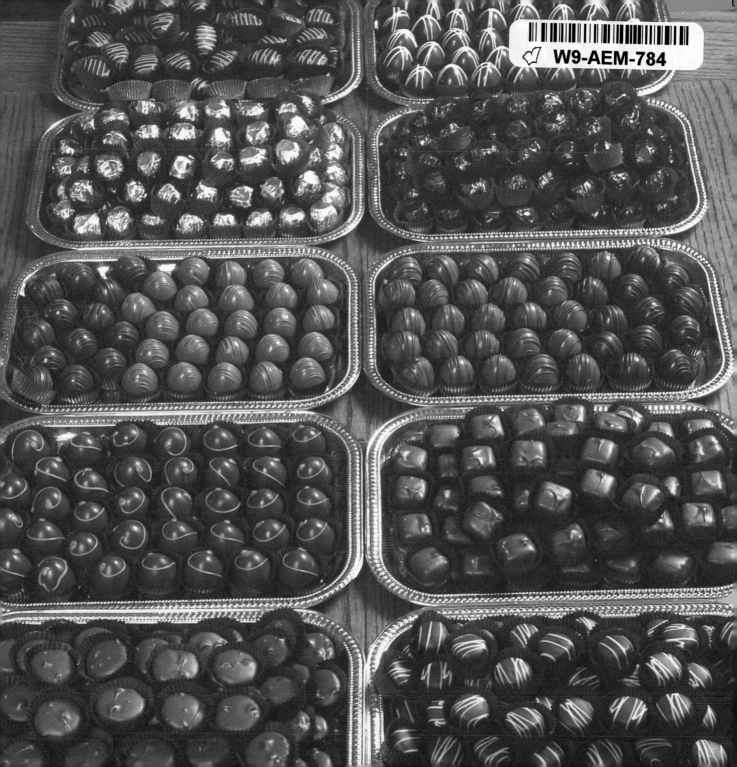

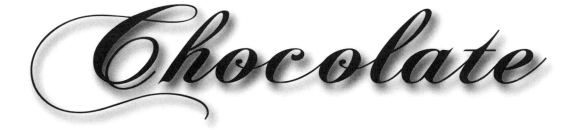

Shara Aaron and Monica Bearden

Chocolate

A
Healthy Passion

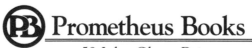
Prometheus Books

59 John Glenn Drive
Amherst, New York 14228–2119

Published 2008 by Prometheus Books

Inquiries should be addressed to
Prometheus Books
59 John Glenn Drive
Amherst, New York 14228–2119
VOICE: 716–691–0133, ext. 210 / FAX: 716–691–0137
WWW.PROMETHEUSBOOKS.COM

12 11 10 09 08   5 4 3 2 1

Library of Congress Cataloging-in-Publication Data

Aaron, Shara, 1975–
    Chocolate : a healthy passion / By Shara Aaron and Monica Bearden.
        p.   cm.
    ISBN 978–1–59102–653–2 (hardcover)
    1. Chocolate—Health aspects. 2. Chocolate. I. Bearden, Monica, 1974– II. Title.

QP144.C46A26 2008
641.3'374—dc22

                                                                    2008026159

Printed in the United States of America on acid-free paper

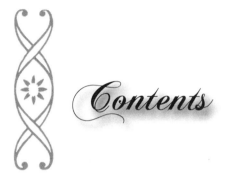

Contents

CHAPTER 5: CHOCOLATE BELIEFS AND TRUTHS 161

Contents

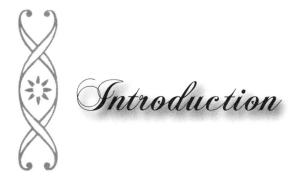

Introduction

The world loves chocolate, and chances are—with 52 percent of the population saying their favorite flavor is chocolate—you do too. This book will serve to deepen your love and understanding of chocolate. Some may think that chocolate is simply a treat, something that satisfies a sweet tooth. After reading this book, you will agree that chocolate is much more than that. You will discover it encompasses a culture, a cuisine, a treatment, and much more! This book speaks to all lovers of chocolate and chocolate connoisseurs by relaying its rich history.

We will first tempt your senses by revealing how to truly savor chocolate. No doubt you already enjoy chocolate, and for this reason you were attracted to this book. We are going to intensify your chocolate experience by teaching you how to get the full chocolate flavor and expand your sensual experience. These skills can be used to impress your friends and family—who will then be forever indebted to you. Next, you will learn how cultures around the world enjoy chocolate; and how chocolate, more than just a flavor, holds a special place in our holidays and celebrations globally. We will also take you on a journey into a rainforest and explore the origins of chocolate. You will learn about cocoa and chocolate coming from a plant that has a friendly relationship with its environment and surrounding communities. We will lead you on an epic journey into the Maya and Aztec cultures, where the chocolate phenomenon began. Through the centuries you will see the transformation of chocolate from a gift from the gods, as revered as gold, to a medical treatment for illness, to a social indulgence for first the elite and, eventually, everyone. We will turn to each part of the story of chocolate in our appreciation of its benefits. Science now proves what was revealed to ancient civilizations so long ago: chocolate does have healing powers. From its potential to prevent illness to its ability to mend a broken heart, chocolate is more than just a pleasurable comfort food—it provides a culture in and of itself.

Throughout the book we include additional special treasures to enhance your love and appreciation of chocolate even more:

> You will find "Chocolate Truffles," which are interesting tips and facts on chocolate, and
> "Cocoa Cravings," which are ancient, traditional, and modern cocoa and chocolate recipes from around the world.

Over the past ten years, chocolate and the food industry together have transformed food into more than just sustenance. The hot news in the media is that dark chocolate is good for you. In the late 1990s we, the authors, began communicating with the media to inform them of the new research on chocolate that showed its potential health benefits. This started the buzz that is so often heard today: chocolate may actually be good for your health! After getting the news out to the public, we next worked with a team to launch the first "Heart Healthy" chocolate brand for a global chocolate company. For the past decade, we have experienced firsthand the excitement of the chocolate phenomenon and are privileged and excited to bring you the true tantalizing story of chocolate.

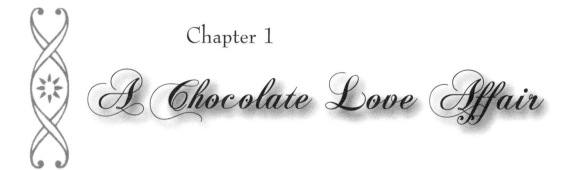

Chapter 1

A Chocolate Love Affair

"Chocolate doesn't make the world go around . . . but it certainly makes the ride worthwhile!"

Unknown

"Research tells us fourteen out of any ten individuals like chocolate."

Sandra Boynton

WHAT IS CHOCOLATE?

Chocolate is everywhere: in our face creams, magazines, news shows, bookstores, and department stores as well as in our coffee, cereals, sauces, and, of course, our favorite treats. Still many may ask, what is chocolate? You might define chocolate in terms of its treats, such as the obvious solid chocolate, but also as chocolate ice cream or any other favorite chocolate dessert. It may surprise you, however, that there is a standard definition for chocolate by the United States Federal Drug Administration that is used by chocolate makers. To be considered real chocolate and not just chocolate flavoring or coating, the product must contain cocoa butter and cocoa liquor (liquid made from ground cacao beans that is very bitter and does not contain alcohol), which are both found naturally in cacao beans.

Real chocolate by US standards cannot contain any other fat besides cocoa butter. Chocolate may contain sugar or other natural sweeteners as well as milk or cream but may not have artificial sweeteners. Other foods may be included such as nuts, fruits, and spices, but the base chocolate must contain at least the first two components found naturally in the cacao bean, cocoa liquor and cocoa butter. This is not necessarily the case around the world where other fats, not inherent in the cacao bean, may be added.

Throughout this book, you'll see the terms *cocoa* and *cacao*, and they're nearly interchangeable, but here's the slight difference: *cacao* refers to the bean, which is the source of chocolate liquor, cocoa powder, and cocoa butter; *cocoa* is the product made by removing part of the cocoa butter and grinding the remainder into a powder. Now that we have our basic definitions down, what about the semisweet versus milk versus baking chocolate lingo? These different types of chocolate contain different ratios of the above-mentioned ingredients (see p. 17 for definitions). Understanding the different varieties of chocolate will not only help you in planning different tastings but will also help you in creating magnificent chocolate recipes.

CHOCOLATE ORIGINS AND BEAN SELECTION

Now that you know the different types of chocolate, we need to bring your attention to the source of the chocolate,

> *Chocolate Truffle:*
> "Extra-bittersweet, bittersweet, and semisweet are all dark chocolates. The difference is the amount of sugar that each contains with extra-bittersweet having the least." (Chocolate Manufacturers Association)

Chocolate 101
(see the color insert for photos of chocolate and cocoa)

Cocoa is made by grinding the remaining part of the bean once you take off the shell and remove part of the cocoa butter. Cocoa can be natural (so nothing is added to it) or Dutch processed (combined with alkali to develop a desired flavor). Both types of cocoa are pretty bitter. In contrast, "cocoa mix" for making hot cocoa has sugar and possibly milk solids added to it. Either natural or Dutch-processed cocoa may be used in recipes; however, highly alkalized cocoa, called "black Dutch cocoa," should not be used in recipes with baking soda because they will interact and produce a soapy flavor.

Natural cocoa has a red-brown color and a fruity chocolate flavor.

Dutch-processed cocoa is cocoa that has been treated with alkali. This reduces the natural acidity, producing a dark brown color and a mellow, mild flavor.

Baking or unsweetened chocolate is pure chocolate—no sugar or milk is added. (For some, their experience with baking chocolate may bring back unpleasant childhood memories of having a very bitter experience after mistaking the big bar of chocolate in the pantry for the expected delight of milk chocolate.)

Semisweet or bittersweet chocolate, both considered dark chocolate, contains a high percentage of cocoa liquor, at least 35 percent, as well as cocoa butter and sugar.

Sweet chocolate, also considered dark chocolate, contains at least 15 percent chocolate liquor as well as cocoa butter and sugar (on the label: typically about 60 percent cacao and up).

Milk chocolate is a combination of at least 10 percent chocolate liquor as well as cocoa butter, sugar, and at least 12 percent milk and/or cream (on the label: typically about 35 percent cacao).

White chocolate is not chocolate because it does not contain cocoa liquor (just the cocoa butter, sugar, milk, and/or cream, and may contain lecithin and vanilla).

the cacao beans (see p. 64 for a photo of cacao beans). Similar to the grapes used to make wine and the beans used to make coffee, cacao beans also vary in aroma, flavor, appearance, and even nutrients based on the region where they're grown. Climate conditions come into play in shaping the characteristics of the beans. The richness of the soil, the amount of rainfall, and the type of trees grown in the various regions influence the dominant "notes" within the cacao bean. (By "notes," we mean the resonant or lasting flavors of the chocolate.) In addition, the way beans are harvested and fermented affects the taste. Like wine, cocoa from around the world is enjoyed for its distinct regional flavor profiles. So distinctive are the differences created by the region as well as the handling of the beans and the making of the chocolate, that tastings encompassing a variety of regions are gaining in popularity. You can choose your chocolate based on the origins of the bean—a truly sophisticated affair.

Below is a guide describing the dominant flavors found in cacao beans based on the different countries where they are grown as well as the different types of cacao beans (source: Hershey's allchocolate.com).

Chocolate Truffle: "Twenty to 50 beans come in each pod and it takes about 400 beans to make one pound of chocolate." (Chocolate Manufacturers Association)

COUNTRY OF ORIGIN

Dominican Republic:

Deep earthy flavor with fragrant tobacco notes

Trinidad and Tobago:

Complex fruitiness and spiciness like cinnamon

Panama:

Classic cocoa flavor with subtle fruit and roasted nut flavors

Venezuela:

Complex fruit flavors like red plums and ripe cherries

Peru:

Slightly bitter with fresh fruity notes

Colombia:

Moderately fruity, lightly bitter, with deep cocoa flavor

Ecuador:

Fruit and well-balanced floral notes

Jamaica:

Bright and fruity, reminiscent of pineapples

Costa Rica:

Fruity with a balanced cocoa flavor

Mexico:

Bright acidity

Indonesia:

Appealing acidity balanced with clean cocoa flavors

Ivory Coast, Ghana:

Deep classic cocoa flavor; lends balance to more complex types of cocoa

Madagascar:

Light citrus flavors, like tangerines, with bright acidity

Truly Tasting Chocolate

To truly enjoy your chocolate tasting, make sure to be in a comfortable and relaxed atmosphere. To begin, take three deep breaths, filling the belly first then the chest. Allow the air to escape slowly, first emptying the stomach and last the chest. This will help release tension and allow you to experience the full satisfaction of the chocolate tasting.

Follow these steps to conduct your own chocolate tasting (adapted from allchocolate.com):

1. Select a sampling of no more than six different chocolates. Any more and your palate's ability to discern the subtle flavor variations will be weakened. Choose what type of tasting you want to conduct (see "Types of Tastings" box, pp. 22–23).

2. Keep chocolate at room temperature, approximately 65–72 degrees F. You want your samples to be at their best. Too warm, and they'll go soft. Too chilly, and it will affect their ability to melt properly and release flavor in your mouth.

3. Each sample should be small. Break your chocolate bars into sections, about one inch by one inch. Really good chocolate is flavorful enough to experience in little bits.

4. Create a plate for each sampling. Include a place card with the name of the chocolate or the original chocolate label for reference.

5. Go from light to dark. Start with milk chocolate, or the chocolate with the lowest percentage of cocoa, and end with the darkest one. This sets up your taste buds correctly to experience the more intense, more complex chocolates as you go along.

6. Once you have the chocolate in your mouth, you will find three distinct parts to savor. First, let the chocolate melt on your tongue for a few seconds to release the primary notes; next, chew the chocolate five to ten times to increase the surface area of the chocolate and to release the secondary flavors; finally, gently push the chocolate to the roof of the mouth and allow it to melt. Notice the feel and flavor of the chocolate. You may even want to close your eyes to block out all distractions and help you focus on just the chocolate.

7. Cleanse your palate between chocolate selections. Water helps clean away the previous flavors. It also quenches your thirst, since some chocolates can leave you thirsty. Water should be room temperature—not ice cold. Very cold water prevents chocolate from melting properly in your mouth and can also dull your taste buds. Dry unsalted crackers and/or plain white bread can also help cleanse your palate. Nibble a bit between samplings, especially after a very strong set of flavors.

8. Jot down your thoughts. If you aim to be a serious chocolate aficionado, consider buying a notebook dedicated to your tasting. Include the date of the tasting, the brand name, and the kinds of chocolates (milk, dark, bittersweet), as well as any other identifying information, if available (region, % cacao, additional ingredients such as vanilla). You may want to create your own rating system, either numerical (1 to 10) or descriptive, such as fair, good, very good, excellent, and superior. Take notes on the chocolate's aroma (sweet, sour, floral); on its texture (velvety, grainy, creamy, waxy); and on its flavor notes and the order of the flavors, since each chocolate will have its very own beginning, middle, and finish. You should also notice how long the flavor lingers and what qualities it leaves behind.

Types of Tastings:

Collection of Percent Cacao: Try a range of chocolates from low, 35% cacao, to high, 82% cacao. You'll be tasting across the gamut of milk, dark, semisweet, and extra dark. In general, the higher the percentage of cacao, the lower the sugar content, which means it becomes more bitter as you go up in cacao percent. The chocolates with the lower percentage of cacao will therefore be the sweeter ones. Start sweet and move to the most bitter, the highest percentage of cacao, so you may experience the most intense chocolate flavors at the end.

Single Percent Cacao: Find different chocolates that all have the same percentage of cacao. For example, taste only 70% cacao chocolates in one session. Note the subtle differences.

Multiple Origin: Sample chocolates from different regions. Observe the variations among chocolates from Central and South American countries such as Guatemala, Venezuela, and Ecuador; or among African, South Pacific, and Asian regions.

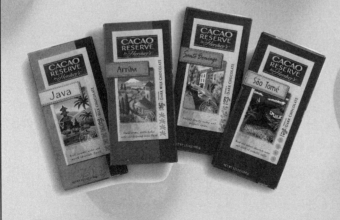

Single-origin chocolate, like Hershey's Single Origin Cacao Reserve bars, offers the opportunity to taste the nuances between various regions' beans. Compare the different flavor notes from around the world.

One Kind of Chocolate: Try a selection of only bittersweet chocolates, or only milk chocolates. Experience the array of aromas, textures, and flavors.

American vs. European Brands: Taste upscale American chocolate bars such as Scharffen Berger and Dagoba, and see how they compare with French and Belgian chocolate bars. All come in different percentages of cacao, and some brands also make variations of flavors from one version.

Filled-Chocolate Tasting: Gather your favorite truffles and chocolate treats filled with almonds, hazlenuts, fresh fruits, or what have you. Let the outer chocolate melt on your tongue first, then enjoy the different textures and fillings. Some fillings may have a hint of saltiness, which helps to intensify other flavors.

Joseph Schmidt, located in San Francisco, California, is an artisan confection company with a line of gourmet truffles, such as Irish cream and peanut butter praline, perfect for a filled-chocolate tasting.

TYPES OF CACAO BEANS

Forastero:

Plain and basic chocolate flavor with low acidity

Criollo:

Complex, fruity flavor

Trinitario:

Range of flavor notes, from spicy to fruity with high acidity

Fortunately, some chocolate manufacturers develop chocolate from one area of origin or that contains only certain beans. By producing bars that have beans from only one region or blends from a few regions, today's chocolate enthusiasts can conduct tastings to identify notes unique to a country or type of bean. To start the process for yourself, pick up a variety of chocolates from different regions and conduct your own chocolate tasting—with friends if you wish.

SUGGESTED WINE PAIRINGS FOR DARK, SEMISWEET, AND BITTERSWEET CHOCOLATE:

Cabernet Sauvignon
Zinfandel
Syrah
Tawny Port
Armagnac
Cognac

SUGGESTED WINE PAIRINGS FOR MILK CHOCOLATE:

Merlot (light bodied)
Pinot Noir
Muscat
Riesling
Sauvignon Blanc
Dessert wines

Courtesy of allchocolate.com and reprinted with permission of the Hershey Company.
© The Hershey Company

Chocolate Truffle:

Chocolate truffles are dome-shaped chocolate confectioneries that can contain all kinds of fillings, including ganache (a filling made from chocolate and heavy cream), flavored creams, melted chocolate caramel, nuts, berries, fudge, nougat, and the list goes on. There are three different types of chocolate truffles: American, European, and Swiss.

- The American truffle is a mixture of dark or milk chocolates with butterfat and may contain hardened coconut oil. Joseph Schmidt, a San Francisco chocolatier, is believed to have created the first American truffle in the mid-1980s.

- The European truffle is an oil-in-water type emulsion and is made with syrup, cocoa powder, milk powder, and fats.

- The Swiss truffle combines melted chocolate with a boiling mixture of dairy cream and butter that is poured into molds then sprinkled with cocoa powder. These truffles must be eaten within days of making—so, if you are eating a Swiss truffle, you know it is fresh.

> **Chocolate Truffle:**
> Chocolate truffles got their name from their resemblance to the highly sought after, edible fungus called the "truffle" used in European cuisine.

TRULY TASTING CHOCOLATE

There is an art and method to truly tasting chocolate. Similar to a fine wine, a chocolate piece must be savored the right way to derive its full satisfaction and enjoyment. It is the different combinations and amounts of natural cocoa butter and cocoa solids as well as the origins and processing of the beans, not to mention any other added ingredients, that can affect the melting and taste properties you are about to experience. A slight variation in the ratios of ingredients and processing can create a whole new sensory experience, including look, smell, taste, and feel. Now, we must warn you, what you are about to learn could possibly make you the most popular person within your social circle. These skills will no doubt create a sense of an underlying indebtedness among your friends and family. The sharing of this enhanced chocolate experience may not only bolster your popularity but also show you are genuinely a good friend.

After you've familiarized yourself with how to do a tasting and experienced the variety of flavors in different types of chocolates, you can invite friends to a group chocolate tasting—perhaps as the finale to a grand gourmet meal. Or pair

> **Chocolate Truffle:**
> "Dark and milk chocolate pair best with red wines. The acidity of champagne or sparkling wines reacts with chocolate, causing a tart taste. Pair these types of wine with white chocolate, instead." (Chocolate Manufacturers Association)

two of nature's most luxurious gifts in one tasting event, wine and chocolate. Thanks to similar components and nuances, chocolate and wine combine very well together. As a rule of thumb, pair dark chocolates with full-bodied reds or rosés and milk chocolates with lighter reds and rosés, some whites, and dessert wines. For a tasting, go from light to dark. Start by swirling, sniffing, then sipping the wine, noting all of the flavors that emerge. Next, take a bite of the chocolate, let it sit in your mouth and begin to melt. Sip the wine again and swirl both together. You'll begin by tasting the fruity acidity, followed by the dominant flavor notes, then a sweet phase, and finally ending with the roasted, slight bitterness of the tannins (bitter and astringent substances found in plants).

HOW TO STORE CHOCOLATE

After your chocolate tasting you may have some chocolate left over. It is very important that the chocolate is stored correctly, so that each time you dip your

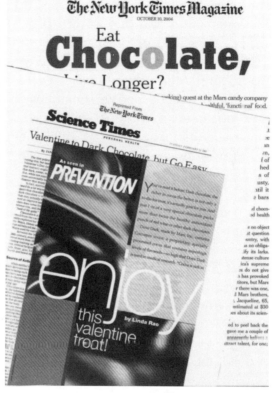

Headlines from magazines and newspapers reporting on the emerging science indicating chocolate and cocoa may have health benefits

hand into the "cookie jar," you get the full satisfaction and flavor that comes with eating chocolate.

Keep your chocolate in a cool and dry place, preferably around 65 degrees Fahrenheit and 50 percent humidity. It does not need to be exact; for example, an air-conditioned room is typically fine.

Store your chocolate in a sealed container to keep it from absorbing other flavors and aromas.

You can freeze chocolate for up to six months. Just make sure to wrap your chocolate in an airtight, sealed plastic freezer bag. When thawing, keep the chocolate in the bag until it has reached room temperature.

A CHOCOLATE LOVE AFFAIR

The world loves chocolate, and based on recent scientific findings, chocolate loves us back. You may have heard the news that "dark chocolate is good for you." This definitely makes for compelling headlines and renders an indulgent and sinful treat not so sinful after all. The inherent tension between tasting great and being healthy has fired up newsrooms and our favorite magazines for the past ten years now. Not only is the news exciting that dark chocolate may have health benefits, but it has lessened our guilt and spurred the "premium" chocolate trend. Dark chocolate sales in the United States went up by 60 percent over the past few years, according to Information Resources, Inc. Similarly, the "premium" chocolate category, including organic, fair trade (helps farmers by guaranteeing fair pricing for their cacao beans), exotic, and spiced chocolate, is growing at a fast pace. Renewed excitement in this age-old category has helped to increase chocolate sales to now a staggering $74 billion worldwide and $17.6 billion in the United States alone (Euromonitor International 2006). So what do these dollar figures mean? In the United States, according to the US Department of Commerce, sales equate to 3.6 billion pounds of chocolate a year. In terms of how much is actually eaten by a single individual, Americans eat 13 pounds a year. The Irish eat the most, 24.6 pounds a year, and the Swiss, a close second, consume 23.5 pounds a year (Euromonitor International 2006).

Mirroring the spread of cocoa through Europe in the 1700s, chocolate is making a resurgence around the world. New regional flavors and bold product launches are spreading the love of chocolate beyond the United States and European nations. Chocolate sales are growing in other countries not typically populated with big chocolate eaters. The Chinese, for example, are switching over from sugar candies to chocolate. In Indonesia—a major exporter of cocoa, but not a country made up of traditionally big chocolate consumers—chocolate is the fastest-growing "impulse purchase product"—meaning that people don't plan to buy chocolate at the store but end up grabbing it on their way out (Euromonitor International 2006). Companies making more chocolate available in these countries is partly the reason for the increase, but the adaptation of chocolate to the regional flavor preferences has also left its mark. A great example of this is found in Asia, where manufacturers have used local flavor as a bridge to introduce chocolate to the population. For example, in China, one of the most popular brands is Le Conté Seduisant Milk & Rice Chocolate, manufactured by Shenzhen Le Conté Foodstuff Co. Ltd., which combines milk chocolate and rice in a bar. In Japan, Nestlé introduced the Green Tea Kit Kat, combining a flavor that already exists within the traditional diet of the area with a well-known global chocolate brand. These types of products are also appearing in the United States

Chocolate Truffle:
"It is believed that molé was created by nuns in Puebla, Mexico, when they combined everything they had in their pantry to satisfy a last-minute visit from an important visitor." (History of Chocolate, Wiley Online Culinary Seminar with Timothy Moriarty, www.pastrywiz.com)

and are considered part of the "premium" chocolate trend.

CHOCOLATE AROUND THE WORLD

Although daily chocolate consumption is growing around the world, chocolate has always held an elite position in many cultures. From bestowing it as a way of declaring love to consoling those in mourning, chocolate as a delicacy is rooted in years of tradition. Various countries and peoples enjoy chocolate as a critical part of celebrations and holidays. In Mexico, Dia de los Muertos (The Day of the Dead) is perhaps the longest-standing celebration including chocolate. Taking place from October 31 to November 2, families build alters to honor their departed loved ones. They leave chocolates, flowers, hot cocoa, or even cacao beans as a gift to the visiting spirits. They eat chicken with chocolate molé sauce (a traditional Mexican sauce made with spices, vegetables, and, yes, chocolate; see recipe on p. 43), and they inscribe the names of deceased family members on the foreheads of chocolate skulls (see color insert for photo of skulls). This custom dates back to the Aztecs, who on the ninth month of their solar calendar would begin a month-long celebration of life and death. The Aztecs believed that life was merely a dream and that in death one awoke. Skulls were displayed as part of the ritual to symbolize death and rebirth. This celebration was seen as sacrilegious by the Spaniards trying to spread Catholicism to the Aztecs. Still, the celebration survived, and today Dia de los Muertos is not only celebrated in Mexico but also by Hispanic populations in certain parts of the United States.

In Japan, Korea, and Taiwan, similar to the United States, Valentine's Day is celebrated on February 14 and makes up 25 percent of the year's chocolate sales. In contrast to the United States, however, it is the women who bestow the gifts of chocolate called *giri-choco* (*giri* means obligation, so "giri-choco" means obligated to give chocolate) to most of the men around them: friends, co-workers, neighbors, and relatives. The special men in their lives receive a more elaborate gift of chocolate called *Honmei-Choco* (*honmei* means "prospective winner," and derives from the courting ritual). These very special Honmei-Chocolates are reserved for serious love. The women spend as much as $200 on the Honmei-Chocolates, which are typically flown in from Europe. Interestingly, among school-aged children, this tradition can be either devastating or uplifting. The popularity of the boys becomes apparent based on the amount of Honmei or Giri chocolate they receive. And some, unfortunately, go home empty handed. For girls, this day is also a day of revelations as they often learn of each other's secret crushes.

In April arrives Easter, the largest chocolate-eating holiday in Australia, with chocolate Easter eggs as the favorite gift. The eggs symbolize new life and are delivered by the Easter Bunny to be eaten on Easter Sunday. A traditional fare during the Australian Easter season is the Hot Cross Bun. A cross symbolizing the death of Christ is placed on top of sweet, spiced buns made with dried fruit and leavened yeast. Recently, a chocolate variation of the Hot Cross Bun has emerged with cocoa added to the dough and chocolate chips replacing the dried fruit (see recipe on p. 45 and photo in the color insert).

The Easter holiday in Germany is also especially rich in chocolate. Many of the customs found in Australia and around the world during this holiday originated in Germany. The Easter Bunny who delivers the chocolates and goodies on Easter Sunday in Germany is believed to have originated as a sign of spring's fertility. It is Germany where the first molded chocolate Easter Bunnies and chocolate-crusted sugar eggs were created (see color insert for a photo of Easter eggs).

In India, late October/early November welcomes Diwali, a five-day Hindu, Sikh, and Jain festival celebrating the triumph of good over evil, inner goodness, and connectedness with reality, as well as praise of the Indian goddesses. Diwali means "rows of lighted lamps" and is often called the Festival of Lights. The lights signify hope for humankind but also remind observers to fuel and strengthen their own inner light. The Goddess Lakshmi—goddess of wealth and prosperity—is also worshipped. Her return welcomed with lights and decorations. During the celebration, neighbors and friends exchange sweets, including chocolate-molded clay lamps decorated with edible paints, chocolate buttons, and flakes in intricate patterns and filled with goodies.

In France, the Christmas Eve dinner is topped off by the traditional Bûche de Noël ("Christmas Log"), a chocolate-frosted cake introduced by a Parisian baker in the 1870s. The origins of this cake can be traced back to an ancient Celtic tradition celebrating the winter solstice, where an actual burning log symbolized the rebirth of the sun. Throughout the years the burning log became more elaborate and was decorated with ribbons and greenery. The youngest to oldest members of the family would set the log ablaze in the hearth to burn throughout the night. The ashes would then be collected the next day and used throughout the year, as they were believed to cure various illnesses, protect the house from storms, and even protect the house from the devil himself. In more modern times the log was turned into a twig, set in the midst of little "friandises" (sweets and delicacies), and eventually, in 1879, into a cake known as Bûche de Noël. The presentation of the cake is the highlight of the French holiday meal (see p. 47 for a recipe and the color insert for a photo of a Bûche de Noël).

A WORLD OF CHOCOLATE CHANGE

Chocolate manufacturers are having a ball making all kinds of gourmet, premium, and exotic chocolates to satisfy consumers' expanding and refined chocolate paletes.

A category that used to be primarily milk, dark, and white chocolate with nuts and dried fruit is expanding to include chocolate made with tea, spices, tropical fruits, and organic ingredients (see the color insert for photos of gourmet and boutique chocolates). In fact, a recent survey by Mintel showed a third of respondents had bought premium chocolate with unusual flavors for themselves in the past three months. Another third said they were interested in trying chocolate with unusual flavors.

THE CHOCOLATE SHIFT

Why such a shift now? Why are we no longer satisfied with just a typical milk chocolate bar? Well, we are enlightened. Science is progressing and we are more aware of how our food affects our health. The media have trumpeted information about the impact of various foods and nutrients on our bodies. Chocolate, in particular, began its makeover in the late 1990s when researchers realized that compounds essential to the development of its aroma and flavor might also affect health. Originally it was information borrowed from the tea industry that began the research into cocoa's healthful compounds. Researchers had been looking at the compounds in tea leaves for quite some time and discovered that certain components in tea had an impact on disease. Studies showed that plant compounds in green tea and even black tea reduced the spread of cancerous cells and affected markers of cardiovascular disease. Interestingly, tea contains similar compounds to those found in cacao beans, which led researchers within the chocolate industry to investigate whether the compounds in cocoa would have similar disease-reducing effects. They found that, in fact, they did.

The news that chocolate may be anything more than a guilty pleasure was not kindly accepted at first. Many researchers, health professionals, and the media were highly skeptical. In February of 2000, CNN ran the headline "Chocolate: A Heart-Healthy Confection?" including the question mark to display the uncertainty and even doubtfulness of the possibility. Warnings were printed in new stories that chocolate is high in sugar and fat, and thus one should proceed with caution. Industry critics bashed confectionery manufacturers for telling such stories. The controversy drew even more buzz, and thus the compelling chocolate story gained momentum and garnered global attention. The underlying passion for chocolate was unleashed as intelligent debates and scientific papers were written weighing the scientific findings against health fears. But chocolate was not the only food being repositioned; cholesterol-laden eggs, high-fat nuts, and wine were also being reconsidered as providing potential health benefits. With the support of science as a strong foundation, critics were silenced and chocolate prevailed. As an ongoing result, it is not uncommon to hear local news report the results of a new chocolate and health study. Out of the news came the development of a whole variety of niche chocolate products, noted for promoting health benefits. Never before for the modern-day world would it be imaginable that taste could be rivaled by health as the reason to choose chocolate.

Some may think it is only the past ten years of research, controversy, and education about the health-promoting compounds in the cacao bean that created the "chocolate shift." But this controversy began long ago in the reverse order as the once-revered cacao bean was transformed into a sinfully indulgent treat. It is only in the past decade that science has uncovered what ancient civilizations knew ages ago: that cocoa has medicinal properties. Returning to its roots in cocoa, the most desirable chocolate has been transformed for many from a light and sweet treat to a rich and bolder dark chocolate.

Riding on the coattails of this good news and in response to this burgeoning desire, manufacturers are pouring dark chocolate into what has been a milk chocolate–dominated America. Not only are new dark chocolate products launched almost every day, touting the inherent "antioxidant" benefits (the ability to diminish dangerous free radicals that can attack your body's cells) of the cacao bean, but a whole new chocolate experience has begun. We are becoming more sophisticated in our tastes.

Perhaps more significant than the availability of information for refining our taste in chocolate is that we all feel entitled to enjoy it—and we will stay that way. When cacao first made its way to Europe, it was an elitist drink reserved for the nobility of Spain, Italy, and France.

Upon reaching England in the 1650s, chocolate became available to anyone who could afford it. In fact, by 1657 a chocolate advertisement was placed in an English newspaper for the first time. Originally having appeal for its medicinal properties, chocolate was now attracting attention for its taste as well. Since then, we as a society have embraced chocolate as part of our special occasions.

Not just for Valentine's Day and social gatherings, chocolate is offered to console our friends, loved ones, or even ourselves. What we may not realize is that not only do we feel entitled to enjoy chocolate but, as originally believed, we also may intuitively reach for chocolate for its health benefits; thus we choose to eat chocolate when we feel happy, sad, or somewhere in between.

The uplifting experience is no longer limited to the act of eating chocolate by oneself or with family and friends. Today, the experience also encompasses the atmosphere of the place where you buy it and where you eat it. The once-hip cocoa houses that opened in Europe in the 1700s are now making a comeback in the form of chocolate boutiques, chocolate bars, and chocolate coffeehouses (see the color insert for photos of an old European chocolate house and a modern chocolate house). Our modern-day chocolate customs are still deeply rooted in our ancestry's elitist desire for cocoa. Still, as members of a democratic society, we feel that all deserve chocolate—and not just once a year for Valentine's Day.

THE MUTUALLY BENEFICIAL RELATIONSHIP BETWEEN COCOA AND THE ENVIRONMENT

Another significant dimension to the chocolate story is its associated environmental and economic benefits. Cocoa growing actually plays an important role in maintaining the rainforest environment and local economies. Through agroforestry—the combination of agriculture and forestry—farmers are able to produce commercially valuable foods and create habitats for wildlife while preserving the rainforest.

Cacao trees are picky; they thrive in

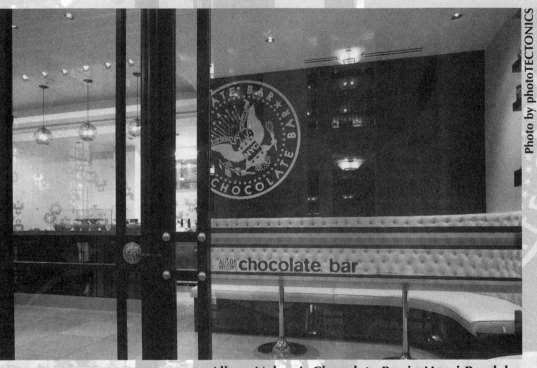

Photo by photoTECTONICS

Alison Nelson's Chocolate Bar in Henri Bendel, New York City; circa 2007. Making a strong comeback, chocolate houses are a new hotspot in cities and towns across the United States. Design by REDDYMADEDESIGN. www.reddymadedesign.com. Used with permission.

constant warmth and plenty of rainfall, at least eighty inches of rain a year, and high humidity as well as shade. Interestingly, cacao trees rely on the shade of other larger trees, not just for blocking them from the sun but also to offer an environment for the insects to pollinate the flowers of the cacao tree so they can grow into cacao pods. With these requirements, they grow only in tropical regions of Africa, Asia, South America, and Central America, within approximately fifteen degrees of the equator. These requirements make them the perfect partner to grow with other economically beneficial trees, such as those that produce bananas, rubber, sapotes (small, brown, and round edible fruit from the marmalade tree), and breadfruit. (See the color insert for a photo of cacao trees growing in the rainforest.)

Many equatorial countries depend on cocoa exports for maintaining their economy—the growing and selling of cocoa feeds the families of small farmers around the world. The traditional labor practices of the small family farm are based on the entire family participating in the growing, collecting, and extracting of the cocoa seeds from the pods in order to make their livelihood. (See the color insert for a photo of a farmer growing cocoa.)

The rapid spread of a fungal disease, "witches' broom," not only devastates the families whose income relies on growing cocoa but also has deleterious effects on neighboring plants and animals, such as the golden-headed lion

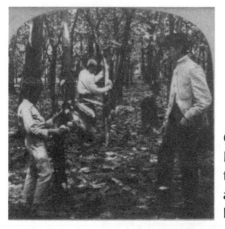

Gathering cacao for chocolate manufacturing, Nicaragua; circa 1903. Traditional farming techniques for beans from centuries past, such as hand cutting pods from trees, remain today. Photo courtesy of the Library of Congress.

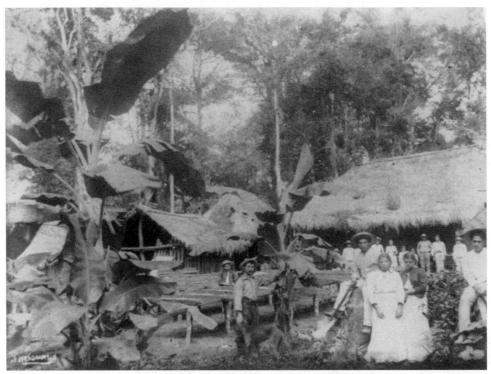

Cocoa plantation between Granada and Leon,
Nicaragua; circa 1900. Growing and selling cocoa has
supported families of small farmers for many decades.
Photo courtesy of the Library of Congress.

Chocolate Truffle:
"Seventy percent of the world's supply of cocoa comes
from a few West African nations, such as the Ivory Coast,
Ghana, Nigeria, and Cameroon." (cocoatree.com)

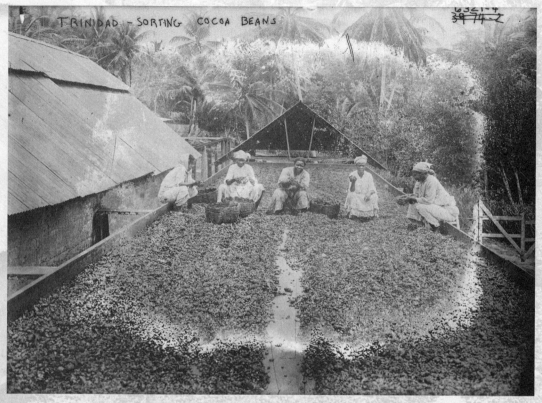

TRINIDAD — SORTING COCOA BEANS

In Trinidad, the women on the farm sort
through cacao beans, discarding those
that are blemished or rotten.
Photo courtesy of the Library of Congress.

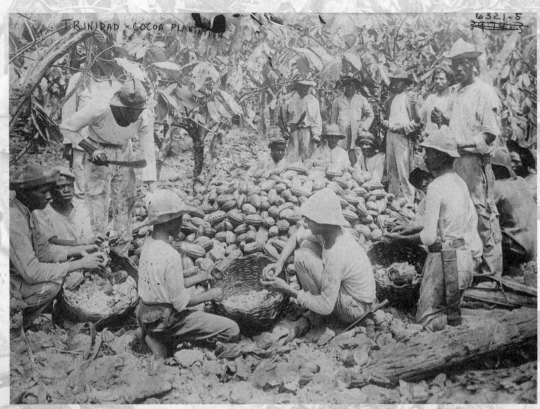

Men and women opening cacao pods on a plantation in Trinidad.
The labor-intensive practice of farming for cocoa production
requires the entire family's participation.
Photo courtesy of the Library of Congress.

> *Chocolate Truffle:*
> "Forty to 50 million people depend on cocoa for their livelihood." (Chocolate Manufacturer's Association)

tamarin monkey. This endangered species lives among the cocoa grown in the shade of southern Bahia's lowland forests in Brazil. Problems with the cocoa crop ravage the livelihood of local farmers, who in turn seek alternative sources of income. By converting these natural habitats into cattle ranches, the golden-headed lion tamarin monkey is in danger of becoming extinct. The *Smithsonian* reports that by saving the cocoa crop from disease through research and developing disease-resistant varieties, the golden-headed lion tamarin monkey and other endangered and endemic species of the coastal forests of Brazil may be spared. Who would have thought that by indulging in your love for chocolate, you would be helping families make a living and supporting wildlife all the way around the world.

> *Chocolate Truffle:*
> "Ten million people live on cocoa farms in West Africa with an average size of approximately 3–7 hectares [7.4–17.3 acres], supporting a family of eight to ten people." (CMA and cocoatree.com)

Cocoa Cravings: Recipes from around the World

Chicken Enchiladas with Molé Sauce

Recipe courtesy of www.allchocolate.com and reprinted with permission of the Hershey Company. © The Hershey Company.

Here's a spin on a traditional dish from Mexico. The sauce is rich with spices that play off the chocolate and make for a flavor sensation.

Ingredients for the molé sauce:

1 tablespoon vegetable oil
2 cloves garlic, minced
1 teaspoon onion, minced
½ teaspoon dried oregano
2½ teaspoons chili powder
½ teaspoon dried basil
¼ teaspoon ground black pepper
¼ teaspoon salt
¼ teaspoon ground cumin
1 teaspoon dried parsley
¼ cup salsa
¾ cup tomato sauce
½ cup semisweet chocolate chips
1½ cups water

Ingredients for the enchiladas:

4 tablespoons vegetable oil
2 pounds skinless boneless chicken breasts, cut into strips
1 medium yellow onion, diced
2 tablespoons chopped garlic
1 teaspoon salt
¼ teaspoon ground black pepper
1 tablespoon ground chili powder
1 tablespoon light brown sugar
1 bunch cilantro leaves, chopped
½ cup chicken broth
5 cups shredded cheddar cheese, divided
20 corn tortillas

Directions for the molé sauce:

1. Heat oil over medium heat in large saucepan.

2. Add garlic; sauté for 1 to 2 minutes.

3. Stir in onion, oregano, chili powder, basil, ground black pepper, salt, cumin, parsley, salsa, tomato sauce, chocolate chips, and water; heat to boiling.

4. Reduce heat to low, simmering for 15 to 20 minutes. Makes about 2½ cups of sauce.

Directions for the enchiladas:

1. Heat oven to 375° F. Lightly grease two 13 × 9 × 2-inch baking pans; set aside.

2. Heat oil over medium-high heat (almost smoking) in large heavy skillet. Carefully add chicken, onion, garlic, salt, and pepper; cook until brown, stirring occasionally.

3. Add chili powder, brown sugar, and cilantro. Deglaze pan with chicken broth. Remove from heat and allow to cool.

4. Pull chicken apart by hand into shredded strips. Stir in 3 cups of shredded cheese.

5. Wrap corn tortillas in damp cloth. Microwave at HIGH (100%) 10 to 20 seconds until soft and pliable.

6. Spoon ⅓ cup (2 oz.) chicken mixture into center of tortilla and roll.

7. Place rolled enchiladas (seam side down) into prepared baking pan.

8. Pour molé sauce over enchiladas. Sprinkle with remaining 2 cups of shredded cheese.

9. Cover; bake 20 minutes. Garnish as desired.

Chocolate Hot Cross Buns
(see color insert for photo)
Courtesy of www.achievesuccess.com.au/easter/easter_recipes.htm

*A delicious take on the traditional
Hot Cross Bun prepared at Easter.*

Ingredients:

1½ cups warm milk
2 packets yeast
Pinch salt
5 cups flour
1 tablespoon cocoa
⅓ cup sugar
1 teaspoon cinnamon
4 tablespoons butter
1 egg, beaten
1 cup chocolate chips
⅓ cup water
4 tablespoons chocolate-hazelnut spread

Directions:

1. Whisk together milk, yeast, salt, and a pinch of sugar in a bowl. Cover with plastic wrap and let sit for 5 to 10 minutes.

2. Mix flour, cocoa, and cinnamon in a large bowl. Add 2 tablespoons sugar, yeast mixture, butter, and egg. Stir until dough comes together. Kneed dough on floured surface until smooth (about 10 minutes). Place in lightly oiled bowl and cover with plastic wrap. Leave at room temperature for 1½ hours until double in size.

3. Punch dough down with fist. Add chocolate chips and kneed until combined. Divide dough into 12 portions and shape into balls. Place in a metal pan (13 × 9) at least 2 inches deep, lined with baking parchment. Cover pan with plastic wrap. Leave at room temperature for 30 minutes until buns double in size.

4. Preheat oven to 400° F. Bake for 20 minutes.

5. To make glaze: Heat water and remaining 2 tablespoons sugar in small saucepan over low heat, stirring until sugar dissolves. Bring to boil for 5 minutes. Brush warm glaze over warm buns.

6. Spread chocolate-hazelnut mixture over buns using zip-sealed bag with corner snipped off.

7. Serve warm or at room temperature.

Bûche de Noël

(see color insert for photo)
Courtesy of Sugar Bakery & Café. Recipe by Stephanie Crocker,
chef at Sugar Bakery & Café, located in Seattle, Washington.

It's best to prepare the cake, filling, and frosting the day before assembling the cake. Once assembled, the cake will keep, refrigerated, for two days; however, the meringue mushrooms must be stored in an airtight container.

Ingredients for the cake:

½ cup all-purpose flour
1 teaspoon baking powder
¼ cup unsweetened cocoa
¼ teaspoon salt
4 egg yolks
½ teaspoon vanilla
⅓ cup granulated sugar
4 egg whites
½ cup sugar

Ingredients for the chocolate mousse filling:

12 ounces good-quality chocolate
3 eggs, separated, at room temperature
3 tablespoons vanilla
1½ tablespoons sugar
12 ounces cream

Ingredients for the chocolate ganache frosting:

12 ounces good-quality chocolate
12 ounces cream

Ingredients for the meringue mushrooms:

2 large egg whites, at room temperature
¼ teaspoon cream of tartar
½ cup sugar
1 tablespoon, approximately, unsweetened cocoa powder
4–6 ounces chocolate

Directions for the cake:

1. Grease and flour a 15 × 10 × 1-inch pan.

2. Sift together flour, baking powder, cocoa, and salt.

3. Beat egg whites until frothy and then gradually add ½ cup of sugar and then continue to beat until stiff peaks form. Set aside.

4. In separate bowl, beat egg yolks and vanilla at high speed 5 minutes until thick and lemon colored, then gradually add ⅓ cup sugar.

5. Fold yolk mixture into whites. Sprinkle flour mixture over egg mix and fold in.

6. Pour gently into the prepared pan. Bake at 350 degrees for 12 to 15 minutes or until cake springs back when lightly touched.

7. Immediately roll into towel dusted with cocoa powder. Let cool.

Directions for the chocolate mousse filling:

1. Melt chocolate over double boiler.

2. While stirring, add the egg yolks and vanilla and mix until well incorporated.

3. Set aside.

4. In clean bowl, beat the egg whites until frothy and then gradually add the sugar, and then continue to beat until stiff peaks form.

5. Fold egg whites into chocolate mixture.

6. Beat cream until stiff peaks form, fold into chocolate mixture, and chill until set.

Directions for the chocolate ganache frosting:

1. Chop chocolate into small pieces and place in quart-sized bowl. Make sure bowl is dry and is not too cold to the touch.

2. Bring cream to boil and pour over chocolate. Stir until chocolate melts.

3. Leave at room temperature about 4 hours or overnight.

Directions for the meringue mushrooms:

1. Preheat oven to 200° F. Line two baking sheets with parchment paper and set aside.

2. Beat egg whites until foamy.

3. Add the cream of tartar and gradually add the sugar until the whites are very stiff and glossy.

4. Load the meringue into a pastry bag fitted with a ¼-inch plain tip.

5. On a baking sheet lined with parchment paper, pipe the caps into even rounds about 2 inches in diameter.

6. Lightly dust the caps with cocoa powder.

7. On a separate sheet, pipe the stems into a cone shape so that the base of the stem is a little broader than the top.

8. Bake the meringues for approximately 1 hour, or until the mushrooms are firm enough that they can be lifted from the baking sheet without sticking.

9. To assemble mushrooms, melt the chocolate over a double boiler or in the microwave.

10. Pierce a small hole in the bottom of each cap.

11. With a small brush, paint the bottom of the caps with chocolate and then insert the stems into the caps.

12. Place on a clean piece of parchment to dry. Store in an airtight container for several weeks.

Directions for the final cake assembly:

1. Unroll the cake and fill with chocolate mousse, and then reroll the cake.

2. Cut the ends of the cake off at an angle to create knots on the "log," which can be adhered to the cake with ganache frosting.

3. To frost the cake, the ganache frosting should be the consistency of corn syrup. If the frosting is too cold, warm it slightly in the microwave, if the ganache is too liquidy, place in the refrigerator and stir often until it reaches the proper consistency.

4. Using a metal offset spatula, frost the cake on all sides, and then use a fork to create the bark texture. Allow to chill 1–2 hours before serving.

5. Garnish with meringue mushrooms and dust with powdered sugar if desired.

Caramelized Pear and Walnut Chocolate Shortcake with Caramel Sauce

Traditional recipe adapted by Shara Aaron and Monica Bearden

Ingredients:

Chocolate shortcake:

2½ cups flour
1 tablespoon baking powder
½ cup sugar
¼ cup unsweetened cocoa powder
½ cup butter, cut into 6 pieces
1¼ cups buttermilk (reduced fat)

Caramelized pears:

3 large pears
3 tablespoons butter
3 tablespoons brown sugar

Caramelized walnuts:

½ cup chopped walnuts
1 tablespoon butter
2 tablespoons dark brown sugar
1 teaspoon vanilla extract

Caramel sauce:

¾ cup butter
1 cup brown sugar
1 teaspoon vanilla
½ cup heavy cream

Directions:

To prepare chocolate shortcake:

1. Grease a large baking sheet with spray canola oil. Heat oven to 400° F.
2. In a large mixing bowl, stir together flour, baking powder, and sugar.
3. Sift in cocoa powder. Stir well.

4. Cut in butter to form a coarse meal.
5. Add buttermilk and mix well. Dough will be soft.
6. Divide dough into six equal amounts and place on prepared sheet. Bake for 20 minutes. Remove from oven and set aside to cool.

To prepare caramelized pears:

1. Wash, peel, and core pears. Cut into thin slices.

2. Melt butter and sugar in a large skillet over medium-high heat.

3. Add pear slices and cook, stirring occasionally until pears are tender and slightly browned on the edges. Remove from heat.

To prepare caramelized walnuts:

1. In a small skillet over low-medium heat, melt butter.

2. Add brown sugar and walnuts, stirring until walnuts are brown.

3. Add vanilla and stir. Remove from heat.

To prepare caramel sauce:

1. In a medium saucepan over medium heat, melt butter.

2. Stir in sugar. Increase heat to medium-high and bring to a boil. Boil, stirring constantly with a wooden spoon, for 5 minutes. Remove from heat and let cool for 5 minutes.

3. Stir in vanilla and heavy cream. (If mixture thickens before using, reheat at medium setting in microwave.)

To assemble:

1. Cut top third off on each short-cake. Set aside.

2. Place bottom of shortcake on individual serving dish. Fan caramelized pear slices over shortcake.

3. Drizzle caramel sauce over pears and on plate.

4. Sprinkle walnuts over caramel sauce.

5. Place remaining tops of short-cakes at an angle on each individual serving dish.

6. Repeat with remaining shortcakes, pears, walnuts, and caramel sauce.

Poires Belle Hélène

Traditional recipe adapted by Shara Aaron and Monica Bearden

Pears poached in vanilla syrup, served with chocolate sauce and vanilla ice cream. This traditional recipe owes its name to Hélène, the queen of Sparta, the principal personnage in the Offenbach operetta La Belle Hélène. *This classic French dessert made its first appearance in restaurants along the grand boulevards of Paris in 1865.*

Ingredients for the pears:

6 firm pears
¾ cup sugar
3 cups water
1 vanilla bean
2 lemons

Ingredients for the chocolate sauce:

8 ounces semisweet chocolate, chopped
½ cup water
1 tablespoon brandy

To serve:

Top with vanilla frozen yogurt

Directions:

1. Peel a pear, leaving the stem intact, and rub immediately with a cut lemon.

2. Working from the bottom, scoop out the seeds and membrane, using a vegetable peeler. Repeat with remaining pears.

3. Pare the zest from the other lemon and then squeeze out the juice.

4. Cut the vanilla bean in half. Combine the water, vanilla bean, lemon zest, lemon juice, and sugar in a saucepan.

5. Heat the mixture until the sugar has dissolved; bring it to a boil.

6. Remove the pan from the heat; add the whole pears. Cut a piece of parchment paper the same diameter as the saucepan. Dampen it and place it on top of the pears to keep them submerged while poaching.

7. Simmer the pears over low heat until tender—about 25 to 35 minutes, depending on ripeness. Let the pears cool in the poaching liquid.

8. Combine the water and chocolate in a saucepan and melt over low heat until smooth.

9. Remove from heat and stir in the brandy. Keep the sauce warm.

To serve:

1. Drain the pears well and place one in the center of each serving plate.

2. Arrange 3 small scoops of frozen vanilla yogurt around the pears.

3. Gently spoon the chocolate sauce over the pears and serve.

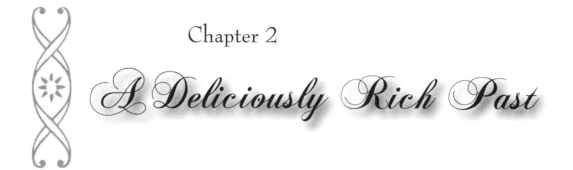

Chapter 2

A Deliciously Rich Past

IN THE BEGINNING

The world's fascination with chocolate began with ancient civilizations dating as far back as 1400–1100 BCE. It is speculated that the first human use of cacao was probably spurred by observing an animal such as a monkey eating the sweet pulp of a cacao pod. This fruit of the pod derives from the plant, the *Theobroma cacao*. At first, people likely discarded the seeds since they are bitter and unpalatable if uncooked. It is believed that the first beverage made from cacao was, in fact, a fermented beer made from the pulp.

An ancient tribe called the Olmecs (1200 to 300 BCE) from the tropical lowlands of south central Mexico was the first known group to bake cacao beans and use them in various recipes, mixing them with the sweet pulp into a concoction called *chica cacao*. Archaeological findings indicate that raw cacao beans were even an integral part of the Olmec diet. They were the first to domesticate the plant and to use the beans they called *kakawa*, or cacao.

Cacao, Cocoa, and Chocolate—What Are the Differences?

All three of these terms are used to describe chocolate.

Cacao = cacao tree or unprocessed cacao beans. This term was used by ancient civilizations and is part of the plant's scientific name, *Theobroma cacao*.

Cocoa = processed beans turned into defatted powder, "cocoa powder," which is also the modern terminology for the plant (i.e., cocoa plantation) and unprocessed beans.

Chocolate = processed beans in liquid or solid form.

For the purposes of this book, *cacao* will be the term used to describe unprocessed beans, as used by ancient civilizations. The drink made from beans will be called *chocolate*, as it is the entire bean in liquid form.

The Maya were the next group to encounter cacao. They are the first group whose relationship with cacao was preserved through artifacts and imagery, showing it to be an integral part of their religion and culture. They preserved the history of cacao through storytelling, images on pottery, stonework, and colorful documents called the codices. It is these documents that have not only helped scientists understand the Maya but have also helped them put together the ancient story of chocolate.

The Mayan territory included the countries we know today as southern Mexico, Belize, Guatemala, Honduras, and part of El Salvador, and existed from 250–900 CE. The Maya likely adopted the terminology and the cultivation of cacao from post-Olmec civilizations,

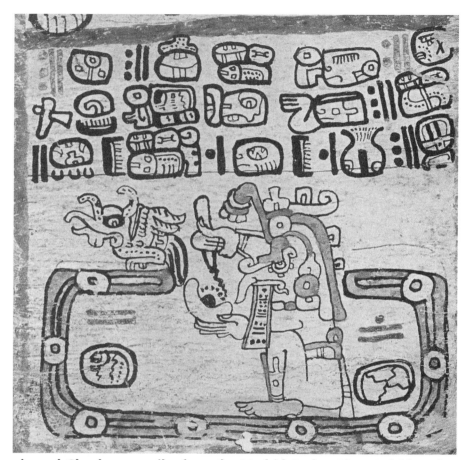

The Mayan rain god Chaak as a scribe from the Madrid Codex. The Madrid Codex contains approximately 250 almanacs that are grouped thematically into sections concerned with the deity Chaak and rain ceremonies as well as planting and agriculture. Throughout the text, the Maya depict the importance of cacao as a crop. Reprinted with permission of Bibliothèque nationale de France.

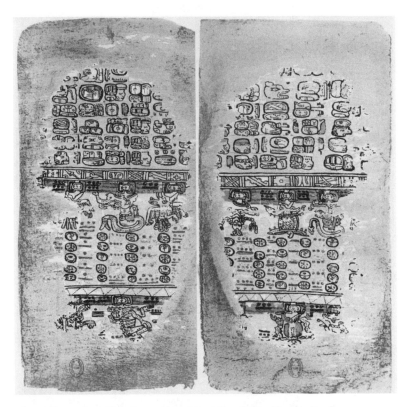

The Maya "zodiac" on pp. 23–24 of the Paris Codex.
Astronomy and astrology were important studies for the
Mayan people, who developed intricate calendars based on the
tracking of the constellations. Tracking the seasonal changes
helped establish their agricultural practices.
Reprinted with permission of Bibliothèque nationale de France.

There are four known Mayan codices that have been named for the cities where they reside: the Dresden, Madrid, Paris, and Grolier codices. The original codices made their way to Europe through different means where they are preserved. The codices can be found in state libraries and museums throughout Europe and most recently in Mexico.

- The Dresden Codex can be found at the State Library in Dresden, Germany. This is the most elaborate of the codices and is believed to have been written right before the Spanish conquest.
- The Madrid Codex resides in the Museo de América in Madrid, Spain, and is believed to have been sent to the Royal Court in Spain by Hernan Cortez.
- The Paris Codex is ensconced in the Bibliothèque Nationale in Paris, France, after being found in a trash can in a Paris library.
- The Grolier Codex was discovered in the 1970s and is said to have been found in a cave. It is not displayed but is kept in a museum somewhere in Mexico. Its authenticity remains in question, however.

began using cacao in ceremonies and as gifts, and incorporated it into their mythology. Such myths are captured in the Mayan sacred book, *Popul Vuh*, which tells their story of creation. According to the *Popul Vuh*, man was created by the gods from plant foods of the Mountain of Sustenance, including cacao. The book also tells a tale in which a cacao tree plays an integral part of the story, illustrating the Maya's high reverence for the plant. It starts with a set of twins born to the old couple who created the universe. In an unfortunate encounter, the twins are beheaded in the Mayan underworld by the lords inhabiting the place— their version of hell. One of their severed heads is hung on a cacao tree. One day the magical head manages to mate with a woman who becomes the mother of twin gods. These two gods in an act of revenge defeat the gods of death who had slaughtered their father and uncle. They rise up to the sky as the sun and the moon to symbolize their act of glory.

The pottery found in actual Mayan burial tombs adds to the mystical story of cacao, depicting offerings for the gods to protect and accept their dead. The pottery also displays hieroglyphics, including images showing cacao drinks being prepared, Mayan gods fighting over beans, and kings waiting to be served cacao creations. These Mayan vessels not only serve as picture books preserved over thousands of years but also provide us with the first physical representation of cacao, which is perhaps the most compelling evidence for scientists of cacao's history. Amazingly, the cacao residues found in the Mayan pottery date back to before 900 CE. It is in these vessels where the Maya stored their precious cacao beans as well as the highly coveted cacao beverage. (See the color insert for a photo of a Mayan vase and ancient pottery.)

The revered drink, or ancient chocolate, was made by grinding cacao beans into a coarse paste and mixing it with spices, water, and chilies to create a variety of hot and cold frothy, bitter drinks. The Maya also mixed it with corn and flavorings to make an assortment of porridgelike meals. Recently, researchers found that the Maya may have even grown cacao in their backyard gardens. In 1976, an ancient Mayan village was discovered in El Salvador where archeologists found preserved cacao seeds in clay dishes as well as the remains of a cacao garden near a Mayan home.

By 900 CE, other groups challenged and took over the empire of the Maya throughout the Yucatan Peninsula. Much of the political power struggle in the region was over who controlled the cacao-rich lands and who had cacao trading

Chocolate Truffle:
The Maya had an extensive trade network, supplying cacao to tribes located in cooler, drier climates that could not grow cacao themselves. (Field Museum 2007)

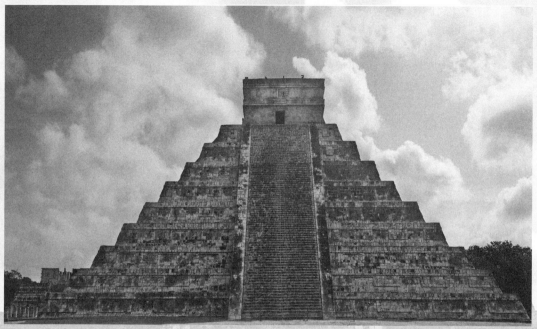

El Castillo in Chichen Itza, Mexico, in the Yucatan was a great Mayan religious center, where cacao played an integral role in ceremony and beliefs. El Castillo is today one of the most visited archeological sites in the world. © Franck Camhi. Image from BigStockPhoto.com. Used with permission.

rights. By 1300 CE, a group of warmongers banded together and took over rule of the region. This marks the beginning of the Aztec reign. As military geniuses, the Aztec people were able to control much of Mesoamerica and elected their first king by 1375 CE. Cacao played a major role in the culture of the Aztec people. Not only were the beans a key trade good, but as the people accumulated wealth, chocolate beverages became a desirable replacement for the native wine.

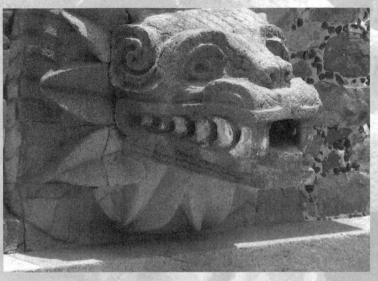

Head of Quetzalcoatl at the temple of Quetzalcoatl in Teotihuacan, Mexico. The god was believed by Aztecs to have given the cacao bean to man and taught them how to cultivate it. © Abigail Gadea. Image from BigStockPhoto.com. Used with permission.

The Aztecs strongly integrated cacao into their rituals and religion. They believed that the god Quetzalcoatl had given the bean to men and taught them how to cultivate it. Quetzalcoatl was banished by the other gods for offering this divinely delicious food to mortals, but he swore to return. (In fact, when Hernan Cortez, the Spanish conquistador, came to the New World in the sixteenth century, the great Aztec king Montezuma believed it was Quetzalcoatl returning.)

Cacao played a role in offerings to the Aztec gods. When slaves were to be killed as sacrifices to the gods, they were served chocolate on the eve of the ceremony to "comfort them." Actual cacao residues have been found at archeological sites where the Aztecs offered chocolate for their deceased relatives.

Chocolate Truffle:
The term "chocolate" is derived from the Aztec Nahuatl language for the word *cacahuatl*, or "cocoa water." The Spaniards then modernized the word to, *chocolatl*. But there may be more to it—the word chocolate seems to be a combination of many ancient words:

Aztec

Choco "cacao"
Latl or *atl* "water"

Maya

Chacau haa/Chocol haa "hot water"
Chocol "hot"
Chokola'j "to drink chocolate together"
Chocol (Maya for "hot") with *atl* (Aztec for "water") = chocolate

ANCIENT CIVILIZATIONS' VERSION OF GOLD: COCOA IN ITS ANCIENT USES

For the Maya and later the Aztecs, money did in fact grow on trees. Cacao beans were the currency of the day. Documents show that the daily wage of a porter in central Mexico in 1545 CE was one hundred beans and the approximate costs of commodities were:

> One turkey = 100 cacao beans
> A small rabbit = 30 cacao beans
> A large tomato = 1 cacao bean
> One turkey egg = 3 cacao beans
> (Coe and Coe, *The True History of Chocolate*, 2006)

The palaces of the kings had warehouses to store cacao beans, which could be compared to today's Fort Knox.

The beans were not only used to pay salaries and other expenditures, they were consumed as a drink by royalty of the palace and those of note. Maya and Aztec people believed cacao was discovered by the gods in a mountain with other wonderful foods. These divine origins were followed with regal uses of

For the Maya and Aztecs, cacao beans were once used as a currency to pay salaries and other expenditures. © Hector Fernandez. Image from BigStockPhoto.com. Used with permission.

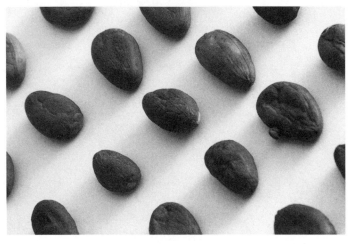

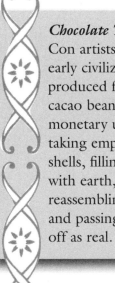

Chocolate Truffle: Con artists of the early civilizations produced fake cacao beans for monetary use by taking empty cacao shells, filling them with earth, reassembling them, and passing them off as real.

cacao, reserved for adult males such as priests, the highest government officials, military officers, distinguished warriors, and sacrificial victims. The chocolate beverage was savored at the end of the meal much like a good port or brandy. However, for the truly elite, cocoa was enjoyed more often. The most famous of the chocolate drinkers was the emperor Montezuma, who drank chocolate throughout his meals, having sometimes fifty cups in a day. Perhaps it is the interesting use of chocolate as an aphrodisiac by Montezuma that started the connection between chocolate and love. It was reported by Cortez and his officer in the early 1500s

Drinking chocolate and other liquids were stored in vessels such as this ancient Mexican jug. © Antonio Ballesteros. Image from BigStockPhoto.com. Used with permission.

that Montezuma would drink chocolate in cups made of pure gold before visiting his wives. Today, current science shows that cocoa and chocolate may improve blood flow. So for Montezuma drinking cocoa could have been invigorating, even producing a natural effect of enhancement prior to lovemaking.

CHOCOLATE MOVES EAST

When Spanish explorers made their way to Mexico in the early 1500s, it wasn't long before they discovered the appeal of chocolate. The first encounter of the Spanish with cocoa is believed to have been when Christopher Columbus and his crew in 1502 captured a canoe that contained strange-looking "almonds," soon recognized as a form of currency in the New World. Although they knew of its use as currency in these regions, the explorers first observed the preparation and consumption of the chocolate beverage in the court of Montezuma. At first, the Spanish as well as other European explorers were repulsed by the bitter beverage, thinking it more appropriate for animal, not human, consumption. Believing the indigenous natives to be savages, the Europeans rejected many of the customs of the New World. Soon after the conquest, in an effort to make this newfound land more like their home, they imported livestock, sugar cane, Old World fruit trees such as oranges and peaches, as well as wheat and chickpeas. These new tastes were forced on the natives. But this was not a one-way street. Living side by side with the Indians induced a change for both groups, and little by little the two cultures began to assimilate. The acceptance of New World practices, specifically the practice of drinking chocolate, by the European for-

eigners is illustrated in the document *History of the New World*, published in 1575 by the Italian explorer Girolamo Benzoni. At first, he described the cocoa beverage as "more a drink for pigs, than a drink for humanity. I was in the country for more than a year, and never wanted to taste it, and whenever I passed a settlement, some Indian would offer me a drink of it, and would be amazed when I would not accept, going away laughing." As time passed Benzoni changed his opinion: "But then, as there was a shortage of wine, so as not to be always drinking water, I did like the others. The taste is somewhat bitter, it satisfies and refreshes the body, but does not inebriate, and it is the best and most expensive merchandise, according to the Indians of that country."

Although we believe it was primarily the men of ancient civilizations who savored chocolate, it may have been the Spanish women in the New World who developed a taste for chocolate first among the new settlers. According to Sophie D. Coe and Michael D. Coe, during an extravagant party in 1538 at the Great Plaza in Mexico City, as recounted by Bernal Diaz in *The True History of the Conquest of Mexico*, the Spanish women were served golden goblets of chocolate. This taste for chocolate among the women may have been influenced by their enslaved Aztec cooks.

In a generation's time, the Spaniards, having a strong sweet tooth, began to sweeten the drink with cane sugar and serve it hot rather than cold or at room temperature. They used spices familiar to them such as cinnamon, anise, or black pepper rather than the Aztec traditional chili pepper, and they created the froth by beating the liquid with a wooden stick called a *molinillo* instead of the Aztecs' custom of "long-distance" pouring (see the color insert for a photo of an Aztec woman pouring chocolate). To help transport the beverage more easily to Europe, the cacao liquor was dried into a wafer that could be instantly turned back into the beverage with water. This "instant chocolate" creation was originally credited to Guatemalan nuns; however, the wafer was really first created by the Aztecs for their military officers. For the next one

hundred years, the Spanish king, nobility, and church officials were able to keep this beverage to themselves. But as the love for chocolate grew in Spain, so did its popularity, such that the "secret" could no longer be contained. Soon, the world would know and demand chocolate.

In the seventeenth century, cocoa made its way to Italy, France, England, and throughout Western Europe. In 1671, the Spaniard Maria Teresa helped fan the popularity of chocolate in France. The new queen, after marrying King Louis XIV, made chocolate popular among the aristocratic women of France, especially among the court in Versailles, by bringing with her Spain's taste for chocolate. To aid them in making chocolate, the French introduced a special pot, called the chocolatiere. The pot had a hinged lid and built-in *molinillo* (called the *moussoir* in French) for frothing the drink, and since the nobility were the primary drinkers, the chocolatiere was made of silver and gold. (See the color insert for a photo of a silver chocolatiere.)

Simultaneous to the arrival of cocoa in France, the English discovered the drink as well. In 1655 England overtook the island of Jamaica from Spain, where cocoa plantations were plentiful, and by 1659 chocolate was available on the mainland. In England, unlike in France, the drinking of chocolate was available to the masses or anyone who could afford to pay for it. Coffeehouses were widespread in England as places where commoners would discuss political issues of the day and chocolate drinks would sit side by side with tea and coffee.

By the end of the seventeenth century, Massachusetts officials were enjoying the chocolate drink. It is unknown exactly when or how cocoa made its way to the new American Colonies, but it is suspected that it was either via the new settlers who came from England or explorers coming from Jamaica.

During the latter part of the seventeenth century or the Age of Reason leading up to the Age of Enlightenment, the foundation for a scientific revolution was unfolding. Physicians and scientists were trying to make sense of the human body and the potential medicinal properties of Mother Nature. Treatises and documents

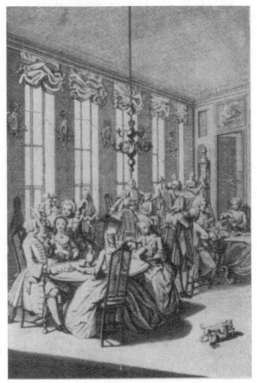

Men and women drinking chocolate in a Liepzig coffeehouse; circa 1700s. At that time thoughout Europe, chocolate was a drink available to the upper crust, who could afford its high price.

were written explaining the relationship between the environment and health. Theories of disease and health as well as tonics made from plants were discussed and debated. Some turned to the impressive ability of the Aztecs to heal with plants and herbs.

FROM MATTERS OF THE HEART TO HEART HEALTH

Interestingly, the popularity and spread of cocoa throughout Europe may have had more to do with health than pleasure. To understand the roots of our current relationship with chocolate in terms of beliefs and passion, we must look back at the development of the Europeans' relationship with chocolate, specifically their original "medical" view of chocolate. To do this, the story once again reverts back to the time of the

Aztec farmers knew the strengths and properties of each and every local plant, as depicted in this page of the Florentine Codex. Reprinted with permission of Biblioteca Medicea Laurenziana.

Aztecs. The Europeans, although they viewed the Aztecs as savages, were obviously impressed with the Aztecs' ability to heal with the use of plants and herbs from the New World. Several documents, the codices, resulted from explorers and physicians trying to make sense of their medical abilities. Chocolate was extensively covered in these documents, which recorded its use to treat many illnesses and conditions. Numerous physicians and authors of the day studied the Aztecs and their customs, and wrote on the medicinal properties of chocolate in its many preparations and forms. The European-

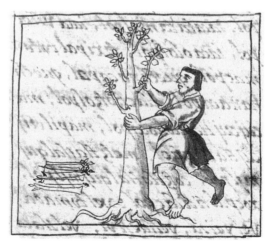

written codices, such as the Florentine Codex and the Princeton Codex, document Aztec customs as well as life in the New World. The Europeans, starting with the Spanish, spent years making sense of what the Aztecs already knew: chocolate had healing powers.

A priest from Spain, Bernardino de Sahagun, who spent sixty years researching and documenting the lives of the Aztecs in *General History of the Things of New Spain*, explained many of the ways cocoa was used to treat illness. It is from this document and the Florentine Codex, written by de Sahagun, that we get an in-depth view and perspective of the Aztecs' everyday lives including their diet, health, and medical practices. Similarly, he also captures the emotional aspect of chocolate that we can still relate to today. He wrote that too many green cacao beans "makes one drunk, takes effect on one, makes one dizzy, confuses one, makes one sick, deranges one. When an ordinary amount is drunk, it gladdens one, refreshes one, consoles one, invigorates one. Thus it is said: 'I take cacao. I wet my lips. I refresh myself.'" Today, we experience many of

the same effects from chocolate as was captured in these original documents. Many of us have experienced that eating small amounts of good, rich chocolate is satisfying and enjoyable and maybe even healthful, whereas too much (well, too much of almost anything) equals indigestion.

The Aztecs' remarkable knowledge also piqued the interest of Philip II in

Chocolate Truffle: When strict and conservative Protestant Pilgrims who fled England for the Netherlands in 1690 took up residence next to a noisy chocolate house in Amsterdam, they became so offended by the ruckus that they dubbed chocolate "Devil's Food." Years later, dark chocolate cakes in Amsterdam were named "Devil's Food Cakes," referring back to the stern Pilgrims.

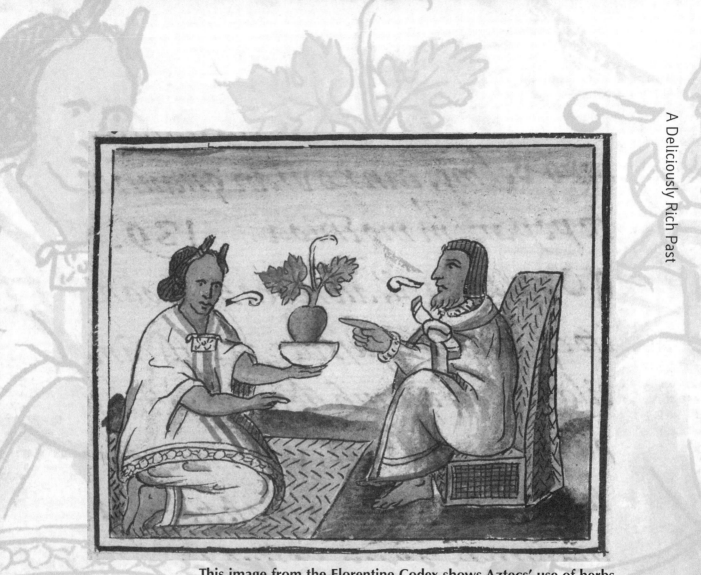

This image from the Florentine Codex shows Aztecs' use of herbs and plants as medicines to heal various ailments. Cacao, in numerous preparations, was used to treat a host of illnesses. Reprinted with permission of Biblioteca Medicea Laurenziana.

Spain. He was so intrigued by the Aztecs' ability to heal and cure with plants that he sent his royal physician, Francisco Hernandez, to the New World in 1570. It is here where he learned of the Aztecs' uses of cocoa to treat stomach and intestinal problems as well as its combination with other plants to cure infection, relieve fever, and dispel faintness. Hernandez wrote that chocolate "warms the stomach, perfumes the breath . . . combats poisons, alleviates intestinal pains and colics."

Not surprisingly, cocoa was also used to mask the bitter taste of other healing herbs and tonics.

Soon other European countries were discovering the healing powers of choco-late. In France and England, there was disagreement on the medical virtues of drinking chocolate, with some believing it a cure-all and others believing its consumption caused illness. The cardinal of Lyon, Alphonse de Richelieu, believed in chocolate's healing abilities and used chocolate "to moderate the vapors of his spleen." But given chocolate's association with the "savages" of the conquered New World, many questioned its efficacy. One English writer, Martin Lister, wrote in his *Journey to Paris in the Year 1698* about his distrust of the new drink, saying that chocolate not only causes corpulence, but that Europeans, unlike the Indians, do not have the ability to digest it, and that drinking chocolate leads to a "worn out, decaying gut." Eventually, as chocolate continued to grow in popularity among the Europeans and in other countries, the debate waned and it was acceptable for physicians to prescribe chocolate to prevent and treat illness. Chocolate was now widely accepted as much more than just a delicious beverage from the New World. The newly formed feelings for chocolate were summed up in 1684 in an influential

Chocolate Truffle: Chocolate was outlawed in the Plymouth Colony in North America by the religious Pilgrims.

document by a French physician and chocolate advocate named Joseph Bachot: "chocolate, well known, is an invention so noble, that it should be the nourishment of the gods, rather than nectar or ambrosia." Almost a century later, chocolate's acceptance by the scientific world was formally set by a Swedish naturalist. In 1753, Carl Linnaeus named the genus and species of cocoa *Theobroma cacao*, or food of the gods. Incredibly, centuries later, the original beliefs of the Maya and Aztec Indians toward cocoa were captured in the nomenclature assigned by this scientist. Through this act, the divine origins of cocoa would not only be preserved in the name, but the potential for further study and medicinal uses would also be established.

Chocolate Truffle: Poisoning used to be a popular method of doing away with your enemies. It is rumored that chocolate was used in Europe to disguise the taste of poison.

It is from these early documents that we are able to ascertain how chocolate was used by the Aztecs and adopted by the Europeans to treat various ailments. As we look at the history of chocolate, you will notice that originally the documentation included not only the physical effects but the emotional as well, as noted by de Sahagun, the Spanish priest. In his opinion, chocolate "refreshes" and "gladdens one." This is not only true for illness and a sense of well-being, but it is also true in matters of the heart.

MATTERS OF THE HEART

It is worth focusing briefly on the customs and writings that set the foundation for the relationship between chocolate and love. Chocolate, love, and intimacy are documented as having both a physical and an emotional aspect. This is apparent throughout the history of chocolate's use, starting with Montezuma's drinking fifty goblets before he visited his wives. The "love" link also had a very clinical aspect, as chocolate was considered by some to be a cure for impotency and an enhancer of fertility and pregnancy. Francisco Hernandez, Philip II's royal physician, wrote that chocolate, "excite[s] the veneral appetite." He included chocolate in recipes to cure impotence. In his treatise on chocolate, Antonio Colmenero de Ledesma stated that "cacao preserved health and made consumers fat, corpulent, faire and amiable." Interestingly, these all were considered positive traits in the seventeenth century and were also believed to help support a healthy pregnancy. His document continued that chocolate "vehemently incites to Venus, and causeth conception in women, hastens and facilitates their delivery." Another text describes how women in labor should be served chocolate. These "love" and fertility beliefs that started with ancient civilizations were then documented by early physicians and still continue today to filter into our modern-day practice of giving chocolate on Valentine's Day. These long-held beliefs, based on theory and testimony, are proving to have real physiological effects as research shows that chocolate may help to keep our hearts healthy and may even have an aphrodisiac effect.

BALANCE AND HEALTH

Despite their vast differences, the Aztec uses of cacao as well as other plants combined well with the European system of maintaining health. The Europeans used a classical Greek–derived system. This system started with a theory developed by Hippocrates around 300 BCE and was refined by a fellow Greek, Galen, born about 130 CE. The Galenic healing system included peculiar ideas, such as using a flower that resembled a human ear to cure an earache. It also contended that magic was linked to astrology. The Aztecs also believed in magic, but as the Europeans witnessed, many of the Aztecs' methods to heal illness using plants and herbs worked. The testimonials of the Europeans helped to preserve the original Aztec uses of cacao, which continued in the post-conquest New World as well as in Europe through today. The New World uses are docu-

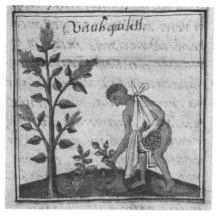

From the Florentine Codex, Aztec healers relied on local plants in the medicinal preparations used for treating and preventing illness. Reprinted with permission of Biblioteca Medicea Laurenziana.

mented as similar to those of the Aztecs in treating kidney disease, liver illnesses, and faintness. The Europeans, impressed by the Aztecs' system of balance, studied their cures and knowledge extensively and incorporated them into the European medical documents.

Both groups believed that health depended on the "balance" of opposites, whereas illness was a result of an "imbalance." For the Aztecs, balance depended on the season, one's age, gender, personality, and exposure to temperature extremes. Also significant was the effect of diet on one's balance. The Spanish in particular focused on "balance" related to "hot/cold" and "dry/wet." Both the Europeans and the Aztecs corrected imbalances by treating the patient with either a complementary or opposite type of food/medicine. So foods and medicines were categorized as either hot or cold, or dry or wet. As the researchers and scientists studied the New World's cocoa, they attempted to assign temperature and humidity classifications for use in medical purposes. Philip II's physician, Hernandez, wrote that the cacao seed is "temperate in nature" as well as "cold and humid." Medical chocolate usually contained anise seed because it helped to neutralize or balance the cold nature of the cacao. In 1591, Juan de Cardenas published a treatise on New World foods in which he classified chocolate as having three very different parts:

"cold," "dry," and "earthy;"
oily, which is "warm and humid;" and
a bitter aspect which is "hot."

Chocolate Truffle:
Casanova, the famous lover, called chocolate his "favorite breakfast dish," revealing in his memoirs that he used chocolate as a bribe for the chaperones and guardians of the women he loved.

He also wrote that chocolate could cause headaches but also aided in digestion and made "one happy and strong." Again, we see that the emotional aspect, happiness, was an appreciated and accepted "medical" effect of eating chocolate. According to Santiago de Valverde Turices, who wrote an extensive treatise in 1624 titled *Un Discurso del Chocolate*, cocoa was "cold" by nature, and when prepared into chocolate was "hot" and "dry" and thus suitable for those suffering from "cold" or "wet"-type illnesses. He also wrote that chocolate was good for the stomach when drunk in small quantities and was good for ailments of the chest when drunk in large quantities.

Chocolate was prepared differently based on the condition to be treated. Among the instructions for treating medical complaints, Hernandez noted that a simple preparation of chocolate, not mixed with other ingredients, was useful in treating fever and infirmities of the liver. But toasting, grinding, and mixing the beans and a gum called *holli* was a preparation to treat dysentery. Another preparation, called *atextli*, which was a thin paste made from cacao beans and maize, was used to excite the sexual appetite. Henry Stubbe, who documented the writings of many authors, botanists, physicians, and travelers in his monograph, *The Indian Nectar*, wrote in 1662 of the many preparations of chocolate in treating various diseases by adding other indigenous plant species to the basic recipe. For example, the flower *xochinacaztli* was added to chocolate to treat weak, phlegmatic stomachs; vanilla was added to the mixture to strengthen the heart and promote digestion; *achiotl* was added to reduce diarrhea, strengthen the gums, or treat a toothache; and *tepayantli* was added to treat cough. Chocolate mixed with Jamaica pepper aided urine and menstrual flow, strengthened the brain, soothed the womb, and dissipated excessive flatulence. According to Stubbe, the basic recipe for medicinal chocolate was:

"To every hundred nuts of cacao . . . put two cods of chile called long red pepper, one handful of anise seeds, and orichelas, and two of the flowers called *mecasuchill*, one vanilla or instead thereof fix Alexandrian roses beaten to powder, two drams of cinnamon, twelve almonds, twelve hazelnuts, half a pound of sugar and as much achiote as would color it."

Physicians were not only creating chocolate "recipes" for health, but they also believed the way chocolate was consumed was very important. Many Spanish physicians wrote and spoke of how to consume chocolate to gain its benefits. The principal physician in colonial Mexico, Dr. Franciscae Ferdinandez, said, "Chocolate is one of the most wholesome and precious drinks that have been discovered to this day . . . very beneficial to our bodies, whether we be old, or young, great with child. . . . And we ought not to drink or eat after the taking of chocolate . . . , nor to use any exercise after it: but to rest for a while after it without stirring. It must be taken very hot." Another physician, Dr. Juanes de Barrios, indicated that chocolate was all that was needed for breakfast because after chocolate, one needed no further meat, bread, or drink.

In a text from 1685 by Sylvestre Dufour titled *The Manner of Making of*

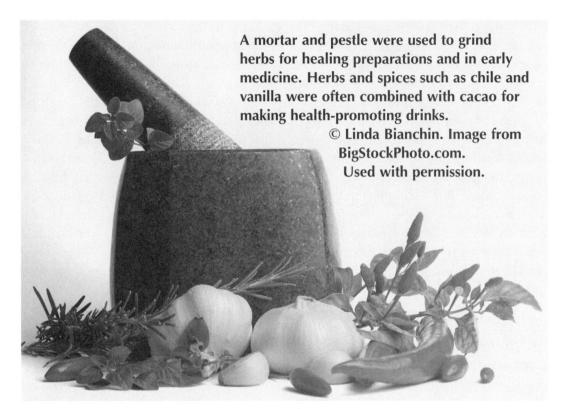

A mortar and pestle were used to grind herbs for healing preparations and in early medicine. Herbs and spices such as chile and vanilla were often combined with cacao for making health-promoting drinks.
© Linda Bianchin. Image from BigStockPhoto.com.
Used with permission.

Coffee, Tea and Chocolate, the author noted that chocolate was a drink of the winter and should be avoided in the dog days of summer.

Numerous other Spanish physicians noted the virtues of chocolate and its ability to not only treat disease but also to sustain health. It was believed that chocolate was instrumental in preserving and prolonging the lives of the Europeans who traveled to the Indies. One author noted that during his time in the region

Historical uses of cacao or chocolate to treat medical conditions		
Anemia	Flatulence	Lung irritation
Asthma	Gout	Nervous distress
Bronchitis	Hangover	Pain
Burns	Heart palpitations	Rheumatism
Cancer	Hemorrhoids	Sexual appetite (promotes)
Colds	Indigestion	Toothache
Colic	Infertility	Tuberculosis
Diarrhea	Insomnia	Tumors
Digestive disorders	Jaundice	Ulcers
Exhaustion	Labor/delivery (promotes)	Wasting/emaciation
Fever	Liver disorders	Wounds

while studying the local vegetation (and partaking in daily chocolate drinks), he had no sick days in over six months. Two other physicians provided this glowing recommendation: "It is the most wholesome and most excellent drink that is yet found out . . . it is good alone to make up a breakfast, needing no other food, either bread or drink, is beneficial to the body, and without exception, may be drunk by people of all ages, young as well as old, of what sex or what constitution so ever and is very good for women with child, nourishing the embryo, and preventing fainting fits . . . preserveth the countenance fresh and fair: it strengthens the vitals." A book from 1719 titled *The Natural History of Chocolate* expanded on the healthful properties of chocolate by discussing its effects on the people of Europe and the Americas in maintaining good health and promoting longevity. It indicated that chocolate was a temperate food, nourishing, easy to digest, and essential to good health. The book went on to discuss the many uses of chocolate in treating illness and then mentioned that "before chocolate was known in Europe, good old wine was called the milk of old men; but since this title is now applied with greater reason to chocolate, hence its use has become so common that it had been perceived that chocolate is with respect to them, what milk is to infants."

From the 1800s on, text after text was published discussing the health properties of cocoa and chocolate, including prescriptive preparations of it as a drink, a food, a topical ointment, and even a suppository. By this time, pharmacists would separate out the oil or cocoa butter and use it for specific purposes such as treating hemorrhoids or as a skin lubricant to heal cracked lips.

By the turn of the twentieth century, chocolate was being mass produced in the form we know it today, as a solid bar. By the early twentieth century discussions of the medicinal properties of chocolate diminished. Instead, chocolate was perceived and eaten more for its pleasurable taste than for its ability to promote good health. (The exception to this is in Central and South America, where people continue to use and believe in the nutritional properties and sacred nature of chocolate. In Oaxaca, Mexico, chocolate is still taken on a daily basis. Sugar, cinnamon, and almonds are added to the cacao beans in the preparation.) It was not until the end of the twentieth century when scientists began looking at the compounds in cacao beans and studying their potential health effects that discussion of chocolate's medicinal properties resurfaced. A shift back to beliefs about its ability to heal and promote health began anew, this time validated by modern-day science. Mother Nature has provided through this tiny bean another example of how food can be the best medicine.

FROM DRINKING TO EATING CHOCOLATE

For much of history, cocoa was used only in drinks—ground up and mixed with various ingredients to be drunk primarily in the medicinal preparations—with the rare exception of its use as an ingredient in recipes. Italian recipes from the late 1600s included cocoa in cakes, pastries, pastas, and meat dishes. In France, cocoa was used in sweets and desserts such as biscuits, mousse, marzipan, pastilles, and creams. The Industrial Revolution of the late 1700s led to many technological advances and a rise in manufacturing and consumerism. From this period on into the 1800s, cocoa evolved from a drink to a food and finally to what we know as today's chocolate bar (as well as all the other delectable chocolate treats). The significant chocolate breakthrough came in 1828 when a Dutch chemist named Conrad Van Houten found a better way to remove cocoa butter to make a powered chocolate. He invented a process that forever changed chocolate production by using a hydraulic press, called the cocoa press. This separated the cocoa butter from the chocolate liquor. What remained was cocoa powder. By "Dutching" the powder, meaning adding alkali to it, not only was it easier to mix but it gave the powder a darker appearance and a milder, less intense flavor. Cocoa powder could then be combined with water to make a chocolate beverage that didn't need complicated mixing or frothing. It was soon produced on a mass scale, boxed, and sold, making chocolate available for everyone.

Once cocoa powder was easy to make, the English Quakers developed the first chocolate bar. In 1847, Joseph Fry, a Quaker, found a way to separate and then blend powdered cocoa with cocoa butter and sugar to make a paste that could be easily molded into a bar. By mixing extra cocoa butter with the cocoa paste, he was able to make chocolate into a portable, solid food. Fry called these new, somewhat crude chocolate bars *Chocolat Dèlicieux à Manger*, or delicious chocolate to eat. All bars previously had to be dissolved in milk or water. This was the very first bar you could eat immediately. Fry quickly became the largest chocolate manufacturer in the world. By the start of the twentieth century, Americans, who were already fond of European chocolates, became interested in producing the treat on domestic soil.

CHOCOLATE IN THE UNITED STATES

Chocolate may have been discovered on this side of the Atlantic, but it took years of refining in Europe before chocolate became the "chocolate" we know today. Thanks to the early confectionery makers in Europe, immigrants, as well as American-born entrepreneurs, the lucrative business of chocolate making was brought to the United States. Many started simply with a dream, ingredients, and a kitchen. Here are some of the stories of the visionary chocolatiers who have helped shape our "chocolate culture."

Ghirardelli

Immigrants to the United States brought their love of chocolate and chocolate-making capabilities with them. Domingo Ghirardelli came to America in 1849 looking for gold but instead went back to his confectionery roots. His San Francisco–based chocolate company, Ghirardelli Chocolate, was built on his years of chocolate experience. Domingo Ghirardelli was born in Rapallo, Italy, where he started his career as a young apprentice to a local candy maker. In 1837 at the age of twenty, he went to

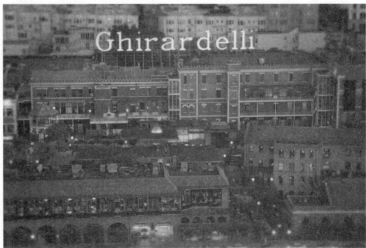

Ghirardelli Square in San Francisco, where the company's chocolate-making facilities resided until 1967. It is now a tourist destination with shops and restaurants. Reprinted with permission of the Ghirardelli Chocolate Company.

Conrad Van Houten invented the cocoa press in 1828, which separates cocoa butter from chocolate liquor and forever changed chocolate production. © Barry Callebaut. Used with permission.

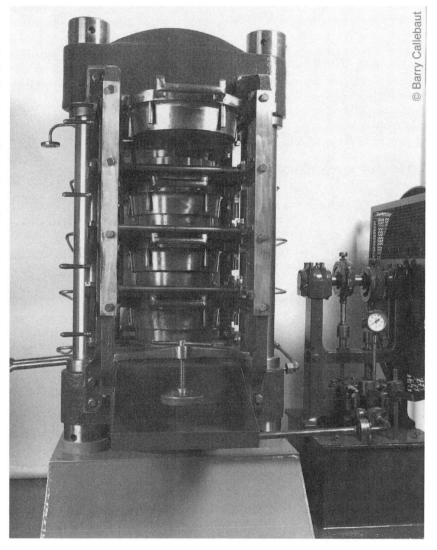

© Barry Callebaut

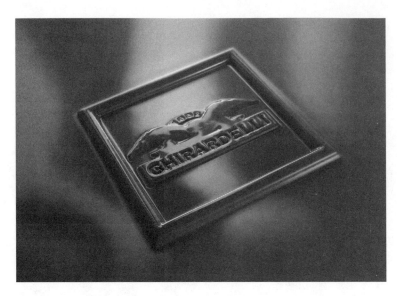

Ghirardelli's signature chocolate square, in solid and filled varieties, has the distinctive seal of the company. Reprinted with permission of the Ghirardelli Company.

Uruguay and worked in a "coffee and chocolate establishment." A year later, he traveled to Peru and opened his first confectionery store. He then made the trip to California in search of gold and settled in San Francisco, where he and his family refined their business ventures. From 1849 to 1900, the Ghirardelli family grew their business, manufacturing chocolate and mustard (who knew?). In 1963 the family sold the company to the Golden Grain Macaroni Company, which in 1986 was acquired by the Quaker Oats Company. In 1998, Ghirardelli was then bought by Lindt & Sprüngli Chocolate out of Switzerland (Ghirardelli.com).

Hershey

After two prior failed attempts in creating a confectionery business, Milton Hershey struck gold with his caramel-making business in Lancaster, Pennsylvania. Soon, Milton Hershey was shipping his caramels all over the United States and Europe. It was not until 1893 that he actually started

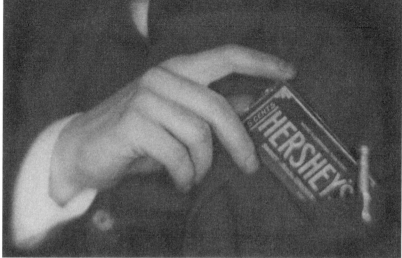

Photograph of an advertisement from the 1920s showing a Hershey's chocolate bar. Photo courtesy of the Library of Congress.

making chocolate. At a chocolate expo in Chicago, Hershey became fascinated with making chocolate. He immediately bought the German chocolate-making machinery from the expo and had it shipped to Lancaster. He then began making chocolate coatings for the caramel sweets he already produced. In 1900, Hershey began producing milk chocolate bars and wafers on a mass scale. This was revolutionary in that it lowered the price and allowed all Americans the luxury of enjoying chocolate, thus locking in the Hershey Company as the All-American Chocolate Company. Adding to this title was Hershey's contribution to our troops starting with World War I, when the company began supplying chocolate as a high-energy food to the military. The Hershey Chocolate Company soon became the biggest chocolate company in the world, producing approximately fifty thousand pounds of cocoa a day by the late 1920s. In the 1940s the Hershey factory was the most modern chocolate-manufacturing facility in the nation, providing more than

Developed in 1907, Hershey Kisses are a signature chocolate product for the Hershey Company. Reprinted with permission of the Hershey Company. © The Hershey Company.

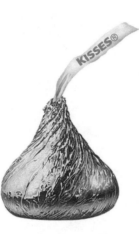

75 percent of the nation's chocolate. In fact, at first, Hershey supplied the Mars family chocolate to make M&Ms and Snickers and Milky Way bars. Adding nuts to chocolate bars and making heat-resistant chocolates that wouldn't melt in warm climates are just some of the innovations Hershey achieved.

As the Hershey Company began to grow Milton Hershey recognized the importance of his workers. He developed Hershey, Pennsylvania, a community created for the welfare of his employees. In Pennsylvania, houses, schools, churches,

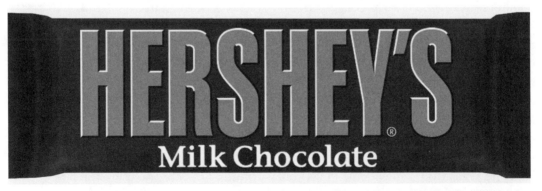

Introduced in 1900, Hershey's famous All-American milk chocolate bar has been enjoyed generation after generation. Reprinted with permission of the Hershey Company. © The Hershey Company.

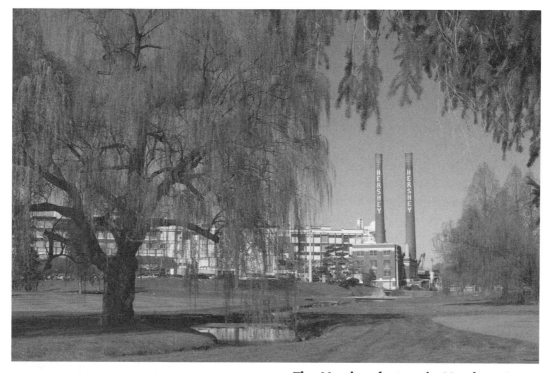

Chocolate Truffle: Bruce Murrie was the son of William Murrie, who was Milton Hershey's right-hand man and president of Hershey for fifty years.

The Hershey factory in Hershey, Pennsylvania, where Hershey's Kisses and Milk Chocolate Bars are made, is just one of the many manufacturing sites for the over-five-billion-dollar company that employs thirteen thousand people worldwide. Reprinted with permission of the Hershey Company. © The Hershey Company.

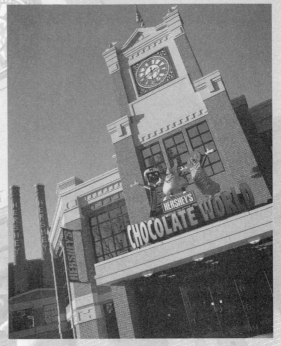

Hershey's Chocolate World is just minutes from the Hershey factory in Hershey, Pennsylvania. Here visitors can take a delicious ride through the fascinating world of chocolate making. Reprinted with permission of the Hershey Company. © The Hershey Company.

parks, and recreation centers were built. Eventually he opened an orphanage for boys, where they would be taken care of and taught technical skills. Although Milton Hershey died in 1945, the town of Hershey and its schools and company continue to grow. Today, Hershey, Pennsylvania, is not only the tranquil home to many of the Hershey Company's employees, but it is also an attraction. Thousands of people visit the Hershey amusement parks for a thrill as well as to sample and buy Hershey chocolate and candies every year. There is even a chocolate spa at Hershey where one can experience chocolate in a whole new way.

Chocolate Truffle:

In 1942 Hershey was ordered by the US military to start full-scale production of the chocolate bar called "Field Ration D" (which would not melt at high temperatures) to feed soldiers in World War II. "The Field Ration D bar was rich with energy and contained 600 calories. The bar was made from a thick paste of chocolate liquor, oat flour, powdered milk, sugar and vitamins and could withstand temperatures of up to 120 degrees Fahrenheit." More than a billion Ration D bars were made the year the United States entered the war against Germany and Japan. An updated version of the technology that kept chocolate from melting at high temperatures was employed to create the chocolate supplied to the troops for Desert Storm. (Hershey.com and *Emperors of Chocolate*)

Scharffen Berger

Scharffen Berger chocolate began as a post-retirement venture for a physician from Mendocino, California. Robert Steinberg, newly diagnosed with a rare form of leukemia, set off to travel through Europe. During his travels he spent time at a small family-owned chocolate maker in Lyons, France. When he returned to San Francisco, he began making chocolate in his kitchen. To develop his idea, in 1996 he partnered with John Scharffenberger, founder of Scharffenberger Cellars champagnes. The two sought to create dark chocolates by using only the finest ingredients. They insisted on quality throughout the entire chocolate-making process, from bean selection to machinery, to achieve the European smooth texture and exquisite taste. Once close to perfecting their chocolate making, the two entrepreneurs sought and secured investors as well as the help of

Scharffen Berger, located in Berkeley, California, uses small-batch artisan manufacturing methods in every step of the process, from roasting the beans to molding the bars. Reprinted with permission of Artisan Confections Company. © Artisan Confections Company.

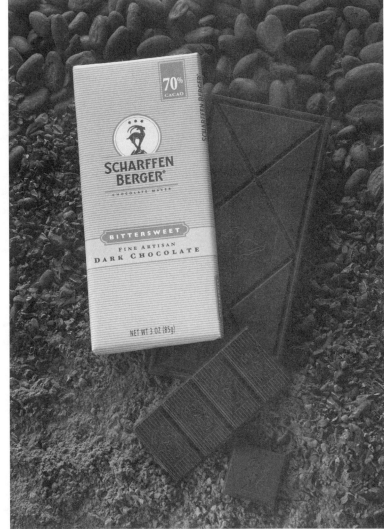

chocolatier Alice Medrich. Having strong support, they proceeded to purchase German chocolate-making machinery and established Scharffen Berger chocolate. By 2001 the company's growth forced them to move into a twenty-seven-thousand-square-foot manufacturing facility in Berkeley, California. Today, Scharffen Berger is owned by the Hershey Company and continues to produce luscious rich chocolates, including a range of high-percentage cacao dark chocolates.

Nestlé

The Nestlé Company started in the 1860s when pharmacist Henri Nestlé developed a formula for babies who were unable to breastfeed. The company began selling the infant formula throughout Europe. Around the same time, a thirty-one-year-old candy maker in Vevey, Switzerland, named Daniel Peter figured out how to combine milk and cocoa powder. The result—the first milk chocolate bar. (Some would argue that it was actually Henri Nestlé together with Daniel Peter who discovered milk chocolate.)

Peter, a friend and neighbor of Henri Nestlé, had started a company—Peter, Cailler, Kohler—that would quickly become a leading maker of chocolate. For three decades the company relied on Nestlé for milk and marketing expertise. In 1929, the almost inevitable merger took place as Nestlé acquired Peter, Cailler, Kohler. Through numerous other mergers and acquisitions, Nestlé is now the world's largest food and beverage company, with annual sales of about $80 billion. Favorite chocolate brands include Nestlé Crunch, Butterfinger, Baby Ruth, and Kit Kat.

Mars, Incorporated

In 1911 Frank Mars and his wife, Ethel, began making and selling a variety of butter-cream candies from the kitchen of their home in Tacoma, Washington. In 1920, after visiting a local drugstore with his son, Frank Mars decided to enter the chocolate-making world. Success came with the Milky Way bar, also called the Mars bar in Europe, which used malted milk as the chocolate center. Interestingly,

Frank Mars was business partners with Hershey and was actually Hershey's best customer. This was not uncommon since, at the time, Hershey supplied the chocolate to most of the nation's confectioners. In the 1930s, Frank Mars's son, Forrest Mars, joined forces with Bruce Murrie to create the M&M Ltd. Company (the first letter of their last names) and chocolate candies.

Forrest's idea for the company and candy came from colorfully coated chocolate candies that had survived the train ride from New York to Hershey, Pennsylvania. This was impressive because no other chocolate could have withstood being wrapped in a napkin inside a pocket for that amount of time. The candy shell provided the chocolate with a protective coating to stop it from melting. M&M chocolate candies soon became a success, and the brand hit celebrity status when M&Ms were adopted as a staple ration for US forces in World War II. Today, Mars, Incorporated, one of the world's largest privately owned companies, boasts an $18 billion business. Other famous Mars chocolate brands include Snickers, Twix, and 3 Musketeers.

Godiva

Godiva Chocolatier was founded in Brussels, Belgium, in 1926 when master chocolatier Joseph Draps founded a chocolate company named in honor of the legend of Lady Godiva. According to the legend, "Hundreds of years ago, a woman of great generosity and beauty left an indelible impression upon the people she reigned over in Coventry. Known for her lustrous hair and bountiful nature, she dedicated her life to the impoverished and stricken. When her husband, Lord Leofric, a powerful ruler, yet unsympathetic to the citizens of his kingdom, imposed a heavy burden of taxation upon his subjects, Lady Godiva protested. Lord Leofric boomed forth a challenge: If Lady Godiva rode naked through the streets, and if the people of the city remained inside, the taxation would be lifted. Lady Godiva agreed to this bet. Although she was demure in spirit, she was always most generous in action. Then finally, it was the morning of the event. Dawn rose, and the clock struck seven, ringing through the cobbled streets. The people closed their shutters, as promised. Lady Godiva's velvet gown dropped to the ground, her luminous skin shimmering. The ride began. Throughout the streets echoed the foreign sound of hooves galloping, yet not a single glance flew her way. Upon her finish, the thunderous cheers were heard throughout the town. Lady Godiva had braved modesty and convention to win the hearts of all who knew her. As promised, Leofric eased his taxation of the poor, and her place in history was immortalized" (Godiva.com).

Centuries later, Joseph Draps, a renowned Belgian chocolatier, created a line of chocolates with extraordinary richness and design, a collection of passion and purity. He sought a name that embodied the timeless qualities of passion, style, sensuality, and modern boldness. Godiva was his choice.

In keeping with the Belgian tradition of elegant, handcrafted arts, Draps introduced Godiva chocolate in his shop on a cobblestone street on Grande Place, selling rich, smooth chocolates. With a focus on detail, he set forth the standard at

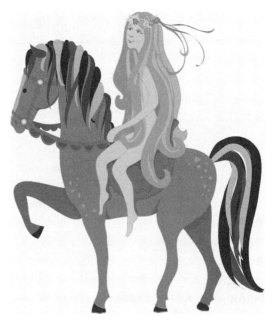

Artist's rendering of Lady Godiva on her horse riding naked through the streets of Coventry. The famous heroine became the namesake of the luxurious chocolatier. © Maria Bell. Image from BigStockPhoto.com. Used with permission.

Godiva for innovative selection of elegant, European shell-molded designs and beautiful packaging. Exquisite European-style gold ballotins, which are special boxes for holding the chocolates, and handcrafted seasonal packaging earned Godiva a reputation for design excellence.

As the success of Godiva Chocolatier grew in Belgium, Joseph Draps sought to expand the company to international horizons. The first Godiva boutique outside of Belgium was opened in 1958 in Paris on the fashionable Rue St. Honoré, followed by openings in the United Kingdom, Germany, Italy, and other European countries. The Godiva brand made its North American debut in 1966, at one of the country's most elegant department stores, Wanamaker's in Philadelphia, Pennsylvania. In 1972, the first Godiva boutique in North America opened on New York's fashionable Fifth Avenue. Today, there are over 275 Godiva boutiques in North America. Godiva is now available in over eighty countries around the world and sold in upscale department stores, boutiques, and mail-order catalogs.

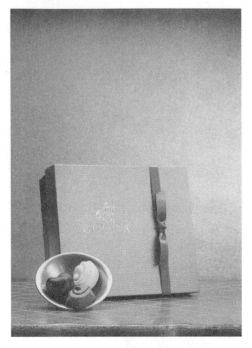

The signature gold ballotin box filled with Godiva chocolates is recognized around the world as a gift of exquisite taste. Photo courtesy of Godiva.

Lindt

In 1845, the confectioner David Sprüngli-Schwarz and his inventive son, Rudolf Sprüngli-Ammann, owners of a small confectionery shop in Zurich, decided to try a fashionable new recipe from Italy for manufacturing chocolate in solid form. The delectable new treat was enjoyed by Zurich's social elite. Production expanded over the next fifty-four years, at which time the company acquired a small but famous maker of chocolate, Rodolphe Lindt, in Berne. The factory was transferred along with the manufacturing secrets and the Rodolphe Lindt brand name to the young Sprüngli Company.

Rodolphe Lindt was probably the most famous chocolate maker of his day. In 1879 he developed a technique by which he could manufacture chocolate that was superior to all others of that period in aroma and melting characteristics. Employing the "conche" (a very important machine to refine and blend chocolate) that he had invented, he produced chocolate with a wonderful delicate flavor and melting quality. His "melting chocolate" soon achieved fame and contributed significantly to the worldwide reputation of Swiss chocolate.

The Swiss chocolate industry, with Lindt & Sprüngli playing a powerful role in this boom, enjoyed great expansion, especially in export markets prior to World War I. With the challenges of the 1920s Depression and World War II, the company's foreign market sales dropped off, yet a quality core business was maintained in Switzerland. Even in difficult times when consumers could hardly afford it, some still wanted only the best of chocolates. From World War II forward, Lindt & Sprüngli enjoyed increased demand for delicious chocolates both at home and throughout Europe. In 1986, Lindt & Sprüngli (USA) Inc. was created, and a manufacturing site and administration building were commissioned in Stratham, New Hampshire. In January 1998, the company acquired the Ghirardelli Chocolate Company of San Francisco, California. Today, Lindt & Sprüngli comprises manufacturing sites in Switzerland, Germany, France, Italy, Austria, and the United States, with Lindt chocolates marketed and sold worldwide to the tune of over $2 billion each year.

Milk chocolate, a favorite in the United States, combines chocolate liquor, cocoa butter, sugar, and milk or cream and contains 35 percent cacao. © *Jostein Hauge. Image from BigStockPhoto.com. Used with permission.*

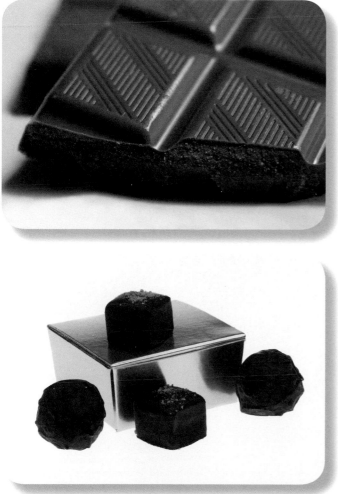

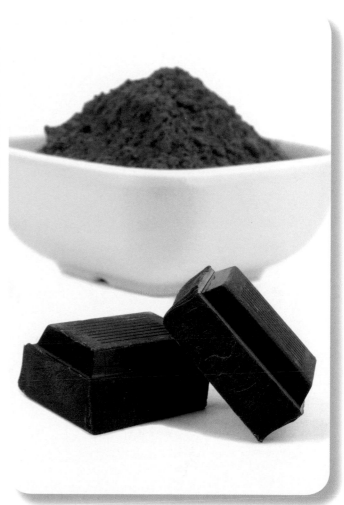

Chocolate truffles are dome-shaped chocolate confectioneries that may contain a variety of fillings, including ganache, flavored creams, caramel, nuts, berries, or fudge. © *Carl Durocher. Image from BigStockPhoto.com. Used with permission.*

Dark chocolate typically contains 60 percent or more cacao—making dark chocolate rich in healthy phytonutrients. © *Norman Pogson. Image from BigStockPhoto.com. Used with permission.*

Chocolate Easter Eggs are believed to have originated in Germany but are now given as gifts and enjoyed around the world to commemorate the Christian holiday. © Timothy Lubeke. Image from BigStockPhoto.com. Used with permission.

Chocolate and candy skulls are used in Dia de los Muertos (Day of the Dead) shrines to commemorate loved ones who have passed. *Photo by Monica Bearden.*

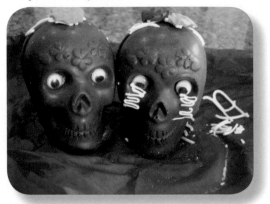

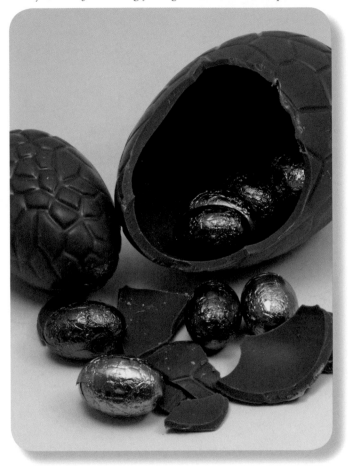

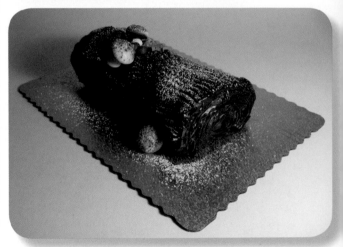

In France, the traditional Bûche de Noël is the grand finale of Christmas dinner. The rolled sponge cake is covered in chocolate buttercream, textured to resemble bark, with smaller pieces of cake, also covered in buttercream, affixed to the main roll to represent trimmed branches. The ends of the roll and the cut faces of the branches are frosted with vanilla cream to imitate cut wood. The log is decorated with holly leaves made of icing or marzipan, and meringue mushrooms. *Reprinted with permission of Sugar Bakery & Café, located in Seattle, Washington.*

A cross symbolizing the death of Christ is placed on top of chocolate Hot Cross Buns, which are made by adding cocoa and chocolate chips to the dough (see recipe on p. 45). *Reprinted with permission of www.achievesuccess.com.*

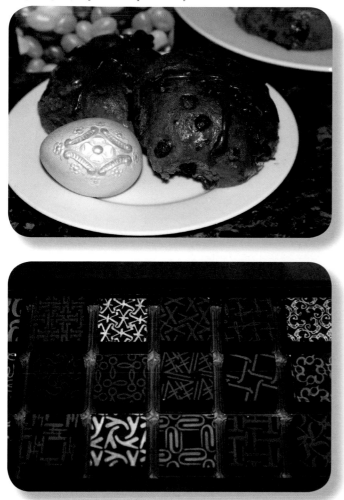

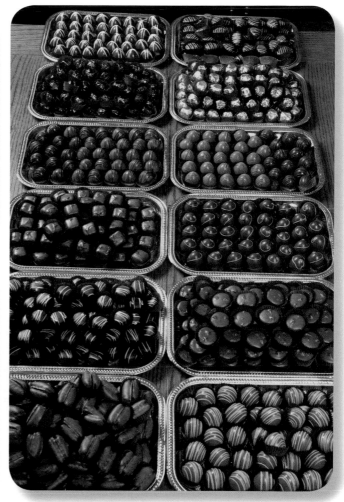

As artistic as they are delicious, designer chocolate pieces are decorated with colorful patterns to please the eye as well as the palate. © *Barak Brudo. Image from BigStockPhoto.com. Used with permission.*

What was once primarily milk, dark, and white chocolate filled with nuts and dried fruit, the gourmet chocolate market has expanded tremendously in recent years to include tea and spiced ganache, tropical fruits, and organic ingredients. © *Mark Stout. Image from BigStockPhoto.com. Used with permission.*

Wealthy men drinking chocolate in a London coffeehouse; circa 1668. As drinking chocolate gained popularity in England, chocolate was the preferred drink in coffeehouses. © *The Trustees of the British Museum. Reprinted with permission.*

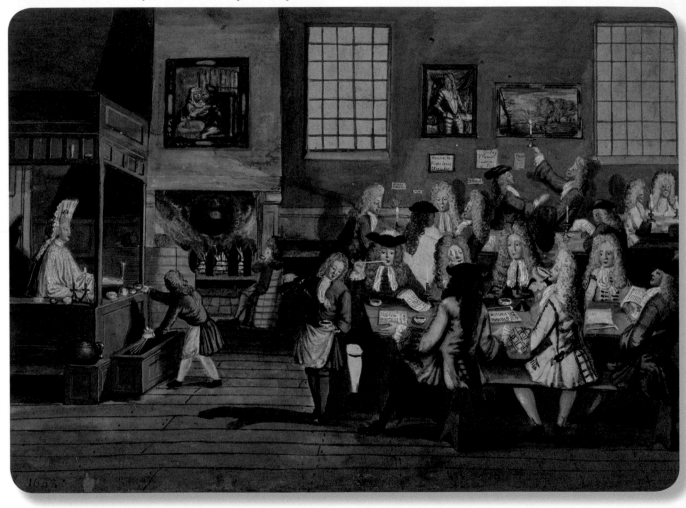

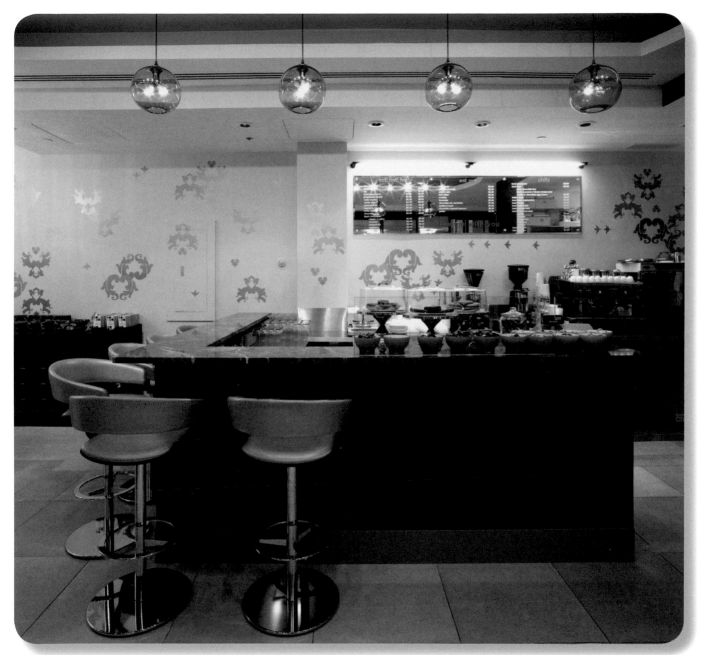

Modern-day chocolate bars offer a variety of treats from traditional sweet drinking chocolate to gourmet, filled chocolates. Today's consumers have a world of choice as compared to their seventeenth-century kin, who originated the gathering place. *Chocolate Bar and Henri Bendel. Photo by PhotoTECHTONICS. Design by REDDYMADE DESIGN. www.reddymadedesign.com.*

This *Theobroma cacao* tree in the Philippines shows the interesting way that the football-size cacao pods grow directly from the trunk and thick branches. *Reprinted with permission of the World Cocoa Foundation.*

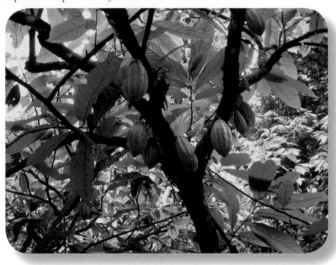

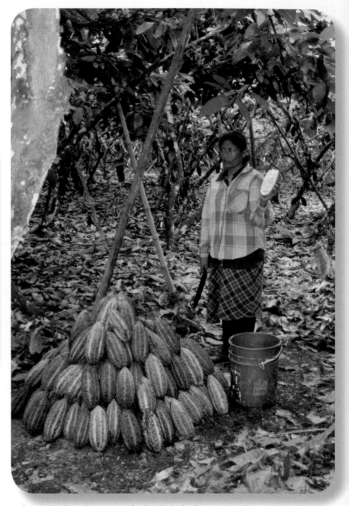

A farmer in Ecuador opens the hard rind of a cacao pod, revealing the white pulp and seeds within. *Reprinted with permission of the World Cocoa Foundation.*

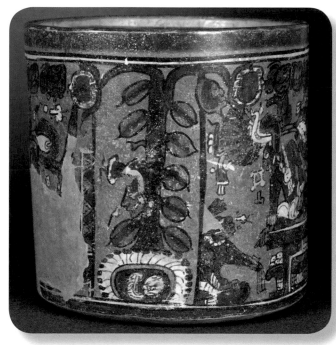

Painting on a Mayan vase, seventh or eighth century CE, Guatemala, depicting the head of the father of Hero Sons hanging from a cacao tree as told in *Popul Vuh. Reprinted with permission of Museo Popol Vul, Universidad Francisco Marroquin, Guatemala.*

The Maya used vases like this one to store cacao beans and a cacao drink made from ground pasta mixed with spices, water, and chilies. © *Rafael Laquillo. Image from BigStockPhoto.com. Used with permission.*

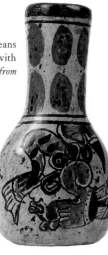

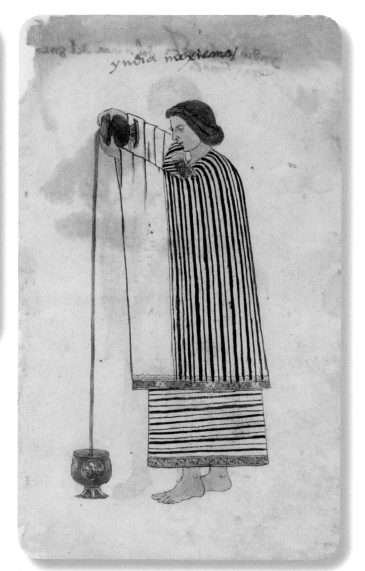

To prepare the drink, the Aztecs, similar to the Maya, ground the shelled cacao beans on a heated metate, or curved grinding stone. They next seasoned the paste with native flavorings such as "ear flower" or chili pepper. They poured from one vessel to another from a height to achieve the froth. They would then drink the beverage cold or at room temperature. From Codice Tudela, sixteenth century. *Reprinted with permission of Museo de América, Madrid.*

An Ulúa-style vase made by the pre-Hispanic Lenca people of northwest Honduras, circa 600–800 CE. Found in the grave of a high-status individual, the vase may have held a chocolately corn gruel or drink consumed during burial rituals. *Photo courtesy of Karla L. Davis-Salazar.*

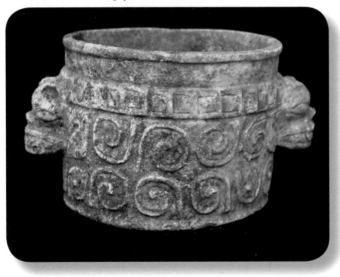

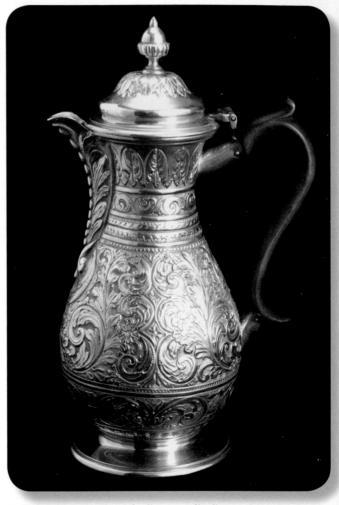

Early chocolate pots, prior to the discovery of kaolin porcelain in France, were typically made of sterling silver and sometimes copper. The earliest pieces included the chocolate stirrer, but later pieces became simply pouring vessels. This silver chocolatiere is from 1852. *Reprinted with permission of the Lincolnshire County Council: The Collection, Art and Archaeology in Lincolnshire.*

Milton S. Hershey, founder of the Hershey Company, circa 1910.

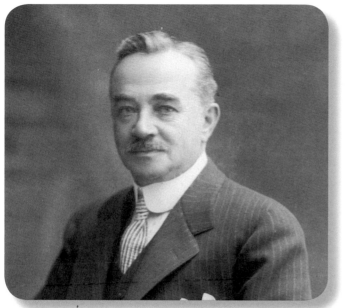

In the late 1800s, the Hershey Chocolate Company was manufacturing 114 different items in all sorts of sizes and shapes, some flavored with vanilla and given luxurious-sounding names to attract consumers. Hershey's Vassar Gems Special Vanilla Chocolate, circa 1896–1909, was marketed to women.

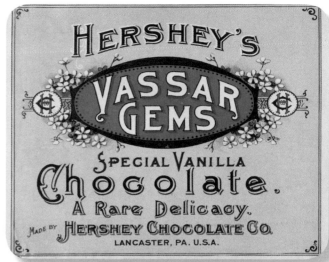

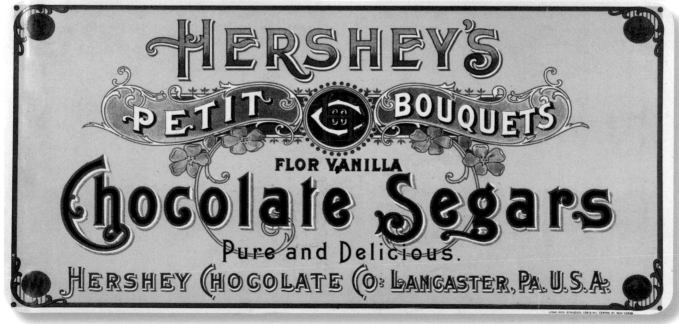

At the turn of the century, chocolate cigars and cigarettes, such as Hershey's Petit Bouquets Chocolate Segars, "Pure and Delicious," circa 1896–1900, were a popular alternative to the tobacco variety.

The original chocolate in bar form was developed by the English Quakers in the mid-1800s. Today's milk chocolate bar is unwrapped and enjoyed by millions. *© Juri Bizgajmer. Image from BigStockPhoto.com. Used with permission.*

Chocolate truffles covered in cocoa powder are filled with flavanols both inside and outside. *© Elena Elisseeva. Image from BigStockPhoto.com Used with permission.*

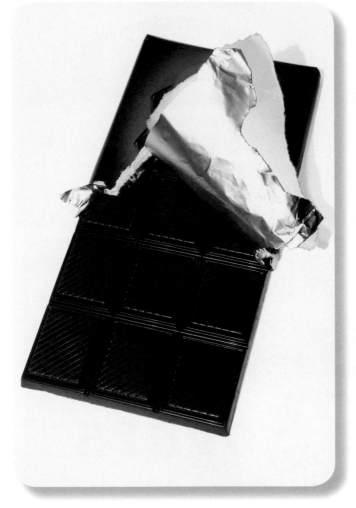

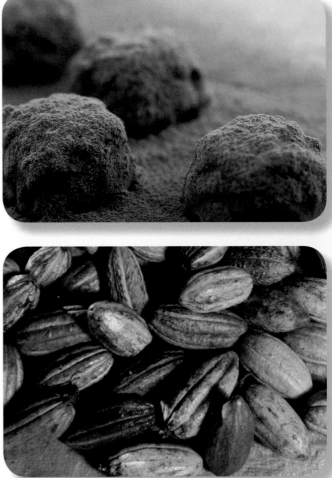

Oblong cacao pods come in color variations such as purple, yellow, orange, and brown. *Reprinted with permission of the Ghirardelli Chocolate Company.*

The thick skin of a cacao pod is sliced open to reveal the sticky white pulp covering the treasure inside—about forty cacao beans. Aztecs viewed the seeds as representing the heart of man. © *David Snyder. Image from BigStockPhoto.com. Used with permission.*

Pods sprout off the *Theobroma cacao* tree. © *Matthew Ragen. Image from BigStockPhoto.com. Used with permission.*

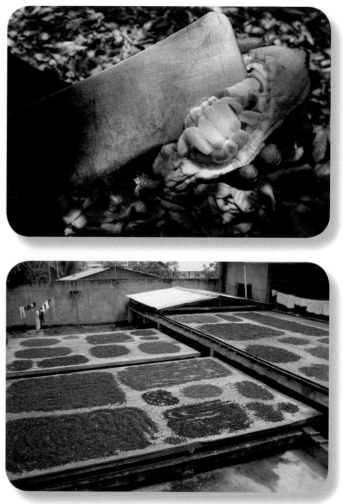

From Ecuador, cacao beans are spread out to ferment and dry in the sun. *Reprinted with permission of the World Cocoa Foundation.*

The process of turning cacao into chocolate starts with the beans. Many companies use a variety of beans from all over the world, which are first sorted by hand. *Amy Snyder, © Exploratorium, www.exploratorium.edu. Reprinted with permission.*

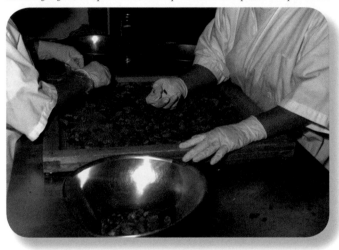

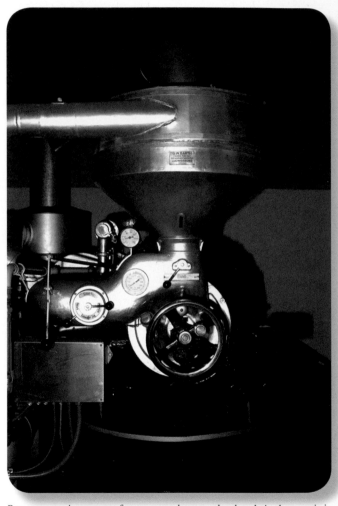

Beans are put in a roaster for up to two hours to develop their characteristic flavor. *Amy Snyder, © Exploratorium, www.exploratorium.edu. Reprinted with permission.*

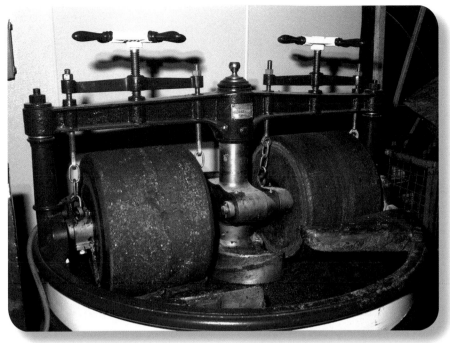

A machine called a melangeur with two solid granite rollers is used to mash and grind the beans, releasing the cocoa butter. After this step, the sugar and vanilla are added to the mix. *Amy Snyder, © Exploratorium, www.exploratorium.edu. Reprinted with permission.*

A concher with rollers that plow back and forth through the chocolate is used to further refine flavor and prolong the mixing process, creating a smooth liquid by coating the cacao and sugar particles with cocoa butter. *Amy Snyder, © Exploratorium, www.exploratorium.edu. Reprinted with permission.*

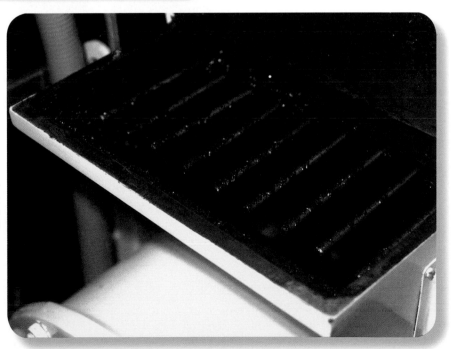

The tempering machine heats, cools, and reheats the chocolate, stabilizing the cocoa butter crystals and giving the finished chocolate a shiny luster and good snap. *Amy Snyder, © Exploratorium, www.exploratorium.edu. Reprinted with permission.*

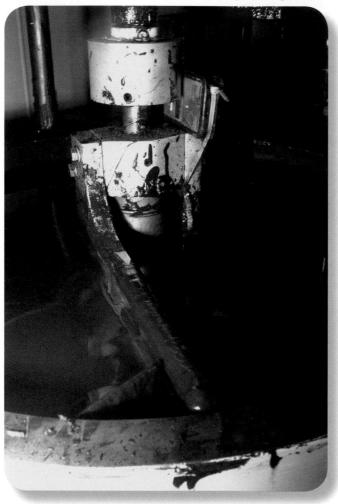

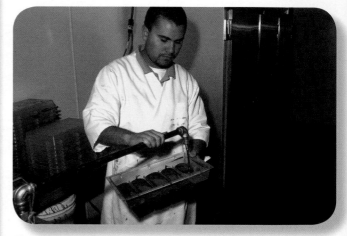

Chocolate is passed through a pipe into a mold. *Amy Snyder, © Exploratorium, www.exploratorium.edu. Reprinted with permission.*

The molds are refrigerated for about twenty minutes to solidify the chocolate. *Amy Snyder, © Exploratorium, www.exploratorium.edu. Reprinted with permission.*

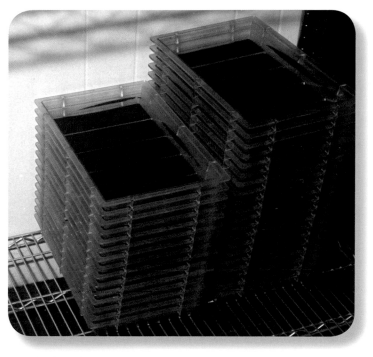

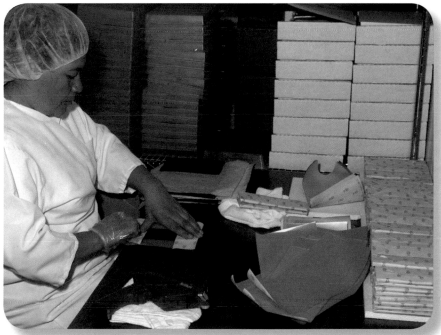

The solid chocolates are then wrapped and packaged for sale. *Amy Snyder, © Exploratorium, www.exploratorium.edu. Reprinted with permission.*

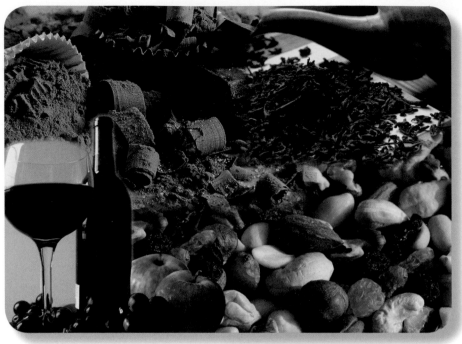

Foods rich in flavanols, such as red wine, tea, and cocoa, may offer potent health benefits. *Photo courtesy of Nutcom.*

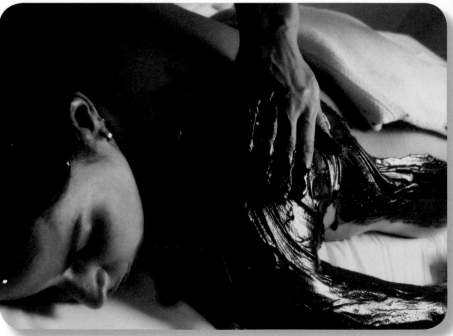

A chocolate massage is one of the new decadent spa treatments that offers a multisensory experience. *© Yanik Chauvin. Image from BigStockPhoto.com. Used with permission.*

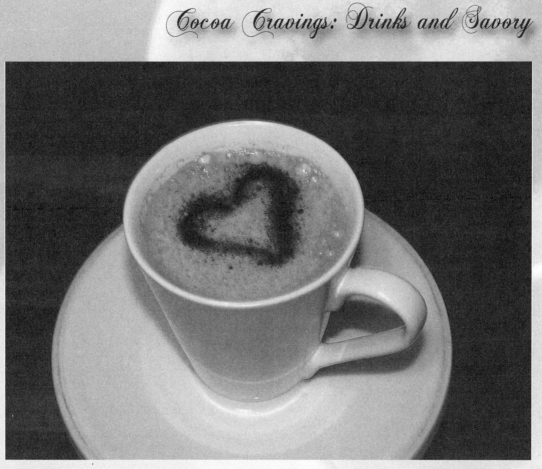

Hot cocoa warms your heart (and may be good for it, too). © Ana Maria Perez. Image from BigStockPhoto.com. Used with permission.

Mayan Hot Chocolate
Traditional recipe adapted by Shara Aaron and Monica Bearden

Ingredients:

2 cups boiling water
1 chile pepper, cut in half, seeds removed (use gloves)
5 cups whole or nonfat milk
1 vanilla bean, split lengthwise
2 cinnamon sticks
8 ounces bittersweet chocolate
2 tablespoons sugar or honey, or to taste
1 tablespoon almonds or hazelnuts, ground extra fine
Whipped cream

Directions:

1. In a large saucepan over medium-high heat, add chile pepper to boiling water. Cook until liquid is reduced to 1 cup.

2. Remove chile pepper; strain water and set aside.

3. In a medium saucepan over medium heat, combine milk, vanilla bean, and cinnamon stick until bubbles appear around the edge.

4. Reduce heat to low; add chocolate and sugar or honey; whisk occasionally until chocolate is melted and sugar dissolves.

5. Turn off heat; remove vanilla bean and cinnamon stick.

6. Add chile-infused water, a little at a time, tasting to make sure the flavor isn't too strong. If the chocolate is too thick, thin with a little more milk.

7. Serve in small cups and top with a sprinkle of ground almonds or hazelnuts and whipped cream.

Makes about 6–8 servings

Espresso Hot Cocoa

Recipe courtesy of www.allchocolate.com and reprinted with permission of the Hershey Company. © The Hershey Company.

Mocha with a serious caffeine kick!
Think of how successful this would have been
in the European coffeehouses.

Directions:

1. In a small heavy saucepan, mix cocoa, sugar, and 2–3 tablespoons of the milk over low heat until ingredients resemble a thick paste.

2. Add remaining milk and stir well, until ingredients are incorporated.

3. Add coffee and heat to serving temperature, stirring occasionally. Do not allow to boil.

Makes about 3–4 mugs' worth

Ingredients:

4 tablespoons Scharffen Berger
    Natural Cocoa Powder, sifted
1 cup milk
3 tablespoons sugar
1 cup strong hot coffee or espresso

Vanilla-Cinnamon Hot Cocoa

by Cleo (Compliments of Chocoholic.com—
your connection to the world of Premium Chocolates)

Ingredients:

4 cups milk
4 tablespoons plus 2 teaspoons
    sugar
4 tablespoons plus 2 teaspoons
    good-quality cocoa powder
¼ teaspoon cinnamon
½ teaspoon vanilla extract
Grated chocolate for topping
A few chocolate chips to melt
    into the mug
Whipped cream or tiny
    marshmallows to float on top

Directions:

1. In a good-sized saucepan, carefully heat the milk (on medium or even medium-high heat) but DO NOT BOIL.

2. Remove from heat, and whisk in the cocoa, sugar, cinnamon, and vanilla.

3. Ladle into mugs, into which you have placed a few chocolate chips, for melting, and then top with the whipped cream (or marshmallows) and dust with the grated chocolate.

4. Stir and enjoy on a cold winter's evening.

Savory Chocolate BBQ Sauce

Recipe courtesy of Ken Gladysz, executive chef of the Hotel Hershey, and reprinted with permission.

Ingredients:

1 tablespoon butter, soft
4 garlic cloves, minced
½ Spanish onion, small dice
2 Roma tomatoes, stem removed, small dice
1½ ounces dark brown sugar
4 teaspoons ancho chili powder
4 ounces apple cider vinegar
8 ounces barbeque sauce
14 ounces vegetable stock
¼ teaspoon cumin, ground
¼ teaspoon cinnamon, ground
⅛ teaspoon cloves, ground
2 ounces Scharffen Berger 82% dark chocolate
2 tablespoons cilantro, fresh, chopped
¾ teaspoon salt
½ teaspoon pepper, fresh ground

This BBQ sauce is reminiscent of the delicious preparations that the early Italians enjoyed on their meat. Made with premium dark chocolate, it has a dark, intense, flavorful taste, with a kick at the end.

Directions:

1. Melt butter in small saucepan over medium heat.

2. Add garlic and onion, sauté 5 minutes until golden brown.

3. Add tomatoes, stir, and sauté an additional 5 minutes.

4. Add sugar and chili powder, mix well, and cook for 5 minutes.

5. Add vinegar, reduce for 5 minutes; mixture should have a paste consistency.

6. Add sauce, stock, cumin, cinnamon, cloves, salt, and pepper. Mix well.

7. Bring to a boil and reduce to a slow simmer for 30 minutes.

8. Add Scharffen Berger chocolate and cilantro; allow to simmer for 5 minutes.

9. Remove sauce from heat and let stand for 10 minutes.

10. Puree sauce, transfer to a clean container, and cool.

11. For best results, refrigerate for 12 hours before using.

Pistachio-Mocha Molé

*by Robert Phillips (Compliments of Chocoholic.com—
your connection to the world of Premium Chocolates)*

Ingredients:

4 5- to 6-ounce boneless
    skinless chicken breasts
1 cup plus 1 tablespoon
    coffee liquor (Kahlua),
    separated
1 cup pistachios, plus extra
    for garnish
1 poblano chile
½ cup chopped onion
3 tablespoons chopped
    cilantro leaves, plus
    extra for garnish
1 tablespoon finely
    chopped bittersweet
    chocolate
1 teaspoon garlic
½ teaspoon chili powder
¼ teaspoon cumin
Salt and pepper
3 cups stock
2 tablespoons cream
1 tablespoon cornstarch

Directions:

1. Trim any excess fat from the chicken breasts. Marinate the chicken in 1 cup of coffee liquor for several hours or overnight.

2. Shell the pistachios, roast them lightly in a skillet, and then coarsely chop them.

3. Carefully roast, peel, and chop the poblano.

4. Preheat a grill or broiler.

5. In a saucepan combine all of the sauce ingredients, except the cream and cornstarch, and bring to a boil. Reduce heat and simmer 30 minutes.

6. Cool slightly. Then carefully pour the sauce into a blender or food processor and puree. Strain through a sieve into a clean saucepan. Mix cream and cornstarch together first, then whisk into the sauce. Heat until slightly thickened.

7. Adjust seasonings to taste.

8. Meanwhile, remove chicken from marinade and wipe off excess marinade.

9. Grill or broil the chicken, turning once, until well browned, about 8 minutes in all. To serve, top each chicken breast with enough sauce to cover and garnish with a sprinkle of chopped pistachios and cilantro leaves.

Yield: 4 servings

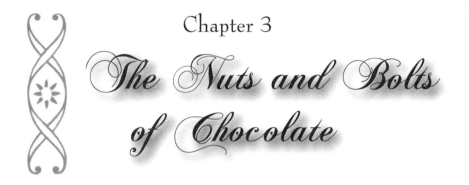

Chapter 3

The Nuts and Bolts of Chocolate

"Chemically speaking, chocolate really is the world's perfect food."

Michael Levine,
nutrition researcher, as quoted in
*The Emperors of Chocolate:
Inside the Secret World of
Hershey and Mars*

Now that we've traced the history of chocolate and its movement across the globe from a medicinal drink to the luscious solid form we know and love today, let's explore how chocolate is actually made and what makes it so amazingly delicious.

Cacao beans come from a tree called *Theobroma cacao*, which grows in certain regions near the equator. By the appearance of the cacao tree, it is hard to imagine that the world's favorite treat starts here. The tree is pretty odd looking. Purplish orange pods in the shape of footballs sprout from the trunk and suspend off the branches. The large pods, which are fruit, look as if they defy gravity. They sometimes jut nearly straight out of the trunk as a single pod or in clusters, or they may hang from the tree's thin branches, dotting the green flora with their colorful fruit. The skin has a thick, rough texture, which almost acts as a disguise to hide the treasure inside. You could say a cacao pod defines the phrase "It's what's on the inside that counts." Once the pod is opened, it reveals about forty cacao beans covered in a sticky, white pulp. Although the pulp is not used in the chocolate-making process, it has already played a vital role in developing the bean's flavor. The pulp tastes both sweet and lemony tart.

> *Chocolate Truffle:*
> A cacao tree must be five or six years old before it will bear fruit. At that point each tree produces about thirty usable pods a year, which translates to roughly one thousand beans total. It takes five hundred beans to make one pound of bittersweet chocolate—so in the best of circumstances, each tree produces beans for only two pounds of chocolate a year.

HARVESTING THE CACAO

Picking the cacao pods, along with most of the steps in cacao farming, is labor intensive. Pods are removed from the tree by hand, using machetes or large knives that are attached to poles to slice down the ripe pods. The workers take care not to damage nearby buds. The pods are then split in half to reveal the pulp surrounding the beans. After scooping out the insides, the outer shell is discarded. If you tasted the beans at this point, they would be extremely tough and bitter.

Once all of the beans are scooped from the pods, they are fermented to continue to develop the beans' flavor. To ferment the beans, they are placed in large, shallow wooden boxes, or piled up and covered with banana leaves. Fermentation starts when the sugar in the pulp is converted to alcohol and then into acids. By changing the chemical composition of the beans, fermentation starts the process of giving chocolate its signature flavor. Enzymes in the beans are activated, which break down the natural sugar and proteins, and generate flavor compounds.

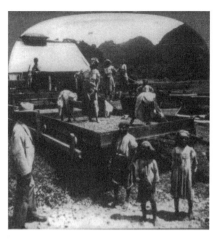

Cacao beans are dried in large, shallow wooden boxes in Dominica, British West Indies; circa 1906. Photo courtesy of the Library of Congress.

Fermentation takes three to nine days, depending on the variety of beans.

When fermentation is done, the cacao beans have a brown color and a fully developed chocolate flavor. This indicates that the beans are ready for drying, a step that removes nearly all the moisture—preserving the beans and preventing mold from growing. There are two ways to dry the beans: by sun drying or by blowing hot air. The best method for keeping the high-quality flavor is to dry the beans in the sun by laying them on bamboo mats for five to seven days. The farmers turn the beans frequently

VARIETIES OF CACAO BEANS
(from allchocolate.com)

There are three main kinds of cacao trees grown throughout the world, all with their own flavor profiles and growth characteristics. There are also hundreds and hundreds of different hybrids of these strains because the cacao tree is quite promiscuous and easily cross-pollinates.

Forastero: Forastero accounts for about 90 percent of all the cacao beans grown in the world. It is prized for its ability to resist disease and its dependability to produce cocoa—making it a favorite of large chocolate producers.

Criollo: Criollo is a flavor bean grown mainly in Latin America. Its susceptibility to disease and low productivity, however, mean many cacao farmers have traded their Criollo trees for hardier plants.

Trinitario: A fusion of the two strains, Trinitario is believed to combine the best of both—good flavor and hardiness. Also considered a flavor bean, it gets its name from the island of Trinidad, where it was first grown.

Chocolate Truffle:
As a general rule, Forastero beans are used as bulk beans, and Trinitario and Criollo beans are used as flavor beans. There are exceptions to that generalization, however. Nacional trees in Ecuador, considered to be Forastero-type trees, produce flavor beans. Whereas, Cameroon cacao beans, produced by Trinitario-type trees and whose powder has a distinct and sought-after red color, are classified as bulk beans.

and pick out any unusable ones. In some regions, such as Brazil, Papua New Guinea, and Indonesia, the climate is humid and rainy, which makes sun drying impossible. In this case, the beans may be dried with mechanical hot-air blowers, which cut the drying time in half. A problem with this method is that chemical reactions started during fermentation are not given enough time to reach completion and may cause the beans to taste acidic or bitter.

After fermenting and drying the beans, farmers take them to collection sites where they are mixed with beans from surrounding farms and loaded into two-hundred-pound sacks. Once the bags are in a central shipping site, buyers can sample the quality of the crop by cutting open sacks of beans to test for proper fermentation. A brown center and aromatic smell indicates a well-processed bean. The beans are then ready to be shipped to chocolate factories and even some small chocolate shops around the world for the next steps in processing—manufacturing the cocoa and chocolate liquor, to ultimately make the chocolate.

Chocolate Truffle:
A hundred years ago, flavor beans accounted for nearly half of all cacao beans. Now they account for less than 5 percent, in large part because the mass production of chocolate in the last century relied on a steady supply of inexpensive beans. However, as chocolate makers produce more upscale products and consumers have learned more about the subtleties and intricacies of chocolate's flavor, the number of flavor beans has been increasing.

FLAVOR BEANS VS. BULK BEANS

The region where cacao beans are grown has an impact on the unique flavor of the beans and ultimately the chocolate. The different tree types also impact the flavor and use of the beans. Some varieties are known as bulk beans and others as flavor beans.

Bulk beans: hearty varieties that make up a good portion of the beans used in making chocolate. They have a classic cocoa flavor. The majority of the beans that come out of Africa are bulk beans from Forastero trees.

Flavor beans: beans known more for their unique taste and high quality. These beans, coming from the Caribbean and Central and South America, provide unique flavor notes to chocolates.

Ecuador is the biggest producer of flavor beans, making more than half the world's supply, approximately seventy thousand tons a year. Other countries growing flavor beans include Colombia, Indonesia, Venezuela, Papua New Guinea, Jamaica, Trinidad and Tobago, Costa Rica, and Grenada.

Many chocolate bars combine both kinds of beans: bulk beans for consistent chocolate flavor and flavor beans for unique tasting notes. But the overwhelming majority of cacao beans produced today are of the bulk variety. Bulk beans are usually less expensive for manufacturers than flavor beans.

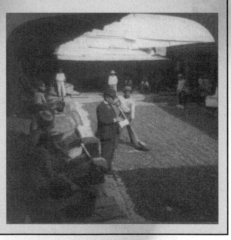

Sorting cacao for shipment to American and European chocolate factories, Guayaquil, Ecuador; circa 1907. Photo courtesy of the Library of Congress.

> *Chocolate Truffle:*
> Cacao beans lose more than half their weight during drying.

TURNING CACAO INTO CHOCOLATE

After making the long journey from Africa, South America, or Central America, the burlap sacks, filled with millions of fermented and dried cacao beans, typically arrive at factories. Some are also delivered to smaller chocolate makers; however, the smaller chocolate shops typically do not start with the beans. Instead, they might receive chocolate liquor, cocoa butter, and crumb—a mixture of chocolate liquor, milk, and sugar—to create their signature chocolates. These beans are now ready to be turned into delectable chocolate bars and cocoa powder. In about one to three days, the bean will be transformed from a tropical seed into the world's most beloved treat. There are ten steps the beans must go through to be transformed into chocolate.

Steps in Chocolate Making

Cleaning: The beans are passed through a machine that removes dried cacao pulp, pieces of pod, and other extraneous material.

Bean roasting: Beans are heated for thirty minutes to two hours at a temperature of 250 degrees Fahrenheit or higher in large rotary cylinders. As the beans repeatedly turn over, their moisture content drops, their color changes to a rich dark brown, and their characteristic aroma of chocolate develops.

Winnowing: The beans are quickly cooled and their thin shells, made brittle by roasting, are removed. A giant winnowing machine, also known as a "cracker and fanner," passes the beans between serrated cones so they are cracked rather than crushed. A series of mechanical sieves separate the broken pieces into large and small grains while fans blow away the thin, light shell from the meat or "nibs."

Milling: Large grinding stones or heavy steel disks crush the nibs. This step begins decreasing the particle size of the cocoa solids closer to that of the finished chocolate. This grinding process also breaks the bean's structure and releases the entrapped cocoa butter, creating enough frictional heat to liquefy the cocoa butter. The result is chocolate liquor (cocoa solids suspended in cocoa butter). The term liquor here does not refer to alcohol. Some of the chocolate liquor goes directly to the blending process and some is pressed.

Pressing: A hydraulic press weighing up to twenty-five tons squeezes much of the cocoa butter from the cocoa liquor, leaving behind solid masses, called "cocoa cakes." These cakes are then pulverized into cocoa powder. The separated cocoa butter drains away through metallic screens as a yellow liquid, which is then collected for use later.

Blending: Ingredients such as cocoa liquor, cocoa butter, sugar, vanilla, and sometimes milk powder are blended in a mixer in various quantities, depending on the type of chocolate being made. The mixture is the consistency of dough.

Refining: The mixture is sent through giant rollers, crushing the chocolate and decreasing the particle size of the cocoa solids and sugar to create the desired finished chocolate effect. This step determines how smooth the chocolate will be.

Conching: A kneading process uses heavy paddles or rollers, depending on the type of conch, to plow back and forth through the chocolate mass. This part further develops the desired flavor by

Chocolate Truffle:
The dry and crumbly result of mixing chocolate liquor with milk and sugar to make milk chocolate is called *crumb*.

> *Chocolate Truffle:*
> Good-quality chocolate typically has a particle size of 25–30 microns and high-end, premium chocolates have a particle size of 15–20 microns. Thus, the smaller the particle size, the silkier the chocolate.

driving off any acidic flavors. It coats the chocolate particles with a layer of cocoa butter and reduces moisture, taking anywhere from a few hours to several days.

Tempering: The chocolate is passed through a machine that heats, cools, and reheats it, thus "tempering" the chocolate. This will ensure that the finished product is glossy, has good snap when broken, and melts smoothly in the mouth.

Molding/Cooling: The warm chocolate is poured into molds of various shapes to make the desired end product: chips, bars, chunks, and so on. The molds are then run through cooling tunnels from twenty minutes to two hours, depending on the size of the chocolate piece, to solidify the chocolate.

Making Cocoa for Baking or Drinking

During the next step, the cocoa butter is pressed out of the chocolate liquor, leaving cocoa cakes. These pressed cakes are then cooled, pulverized, and sifted into cocoa powder. At this point, the cocoa may be "Dutched," or treated with an alkali, to develop a slightly milder flavor and to give the cocoa a darker appearance. A good example of a "Dutched" chocolate flavor is the signature Oreo Cookie flavor.

A WALK WITH WILLIE WONKA

Now that you know the steps involved in making chocolate, we want to lead you through a visual journey inside a chocolate factory. We have been in many chocolate factories around the world and have never been disappointed. At first, the factory may seem unimpressive and very industrial. There are big metal machines, conveyor belts, a lot of noise, and people wearing hair nets and uniforms (sorry, we have never seen any Oompa Lumpas running around). We must admit, before entering our first chocolate factory, we were half expecting to see chocolate rivers and joyful people singing in harmony as they made chocolate. Unfortunately, this was not the case; however, as you look more closely, you do find magic and experience awe in watching the assembly-line creation of chocolate candy.

The beans are delivered in large sacks, which are dumped into a depository near a loading dock. There the beans are cleaned and then fed into a huge oven-looking machine. On the other end, the beans come out toasty and you begin to smell a burnt chocolatelike aroma. Next, these dark brown little beauties are deshelled into nibs. You can eat them now, although they are really bitter and taste, at least in our opinion, nothing like chocolate yet.

Then, depending on the factory, the nibs race up a conveyor belt (they really do look like they are in a hurry) for grinding. At this point, you are well into the main area of the factory and will see several levels, with all kinds of machinery above and below you (gravity comes in handy, helping to transport chocolate from one step to the next). You can see all kinds of machines connected by pipes

Chocolate Truffle:
Growing up on a ranch in Mexico that grew cacao trees, my mom and her sisters and brother used to eat cacao beans raw. This was a common practice in her town where cacao trees flourished.
—Monica Bearden

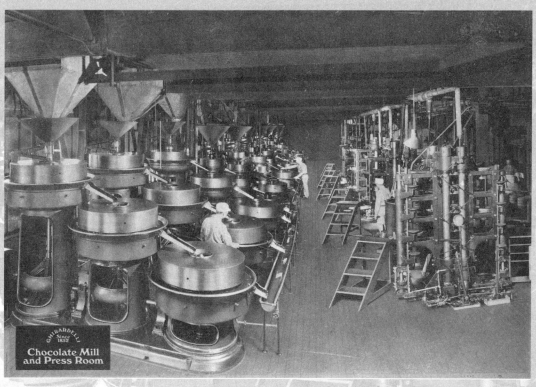

Chocolate Mill and Press Room

Inside the Ghirardelli chocolate mill and press room, where cocoa nibs are ground to chocolate liquor and pressed, removing the cocoa butter and becoming cocoa cakes. Reprinted with permission of the Ghirardelli Chocolate Company.

and conveyor belts in small rooms and big rooms throughout the factory. Throughout these rooms, technicians and engineers make sure that the machines are working correctly. Samples are taken on schedule to the food scientists who are in a lab nearby to make certain that the desired product is being produced in each step. As you are taking all of this in, the hurried nibs are entering into the grinders. This results in a dark and shiny liquid, the chocolate liquor, which is taken by pipes to its next destination. At this point the path diverges. A portion of the rich and silky chocolate goes to a very ominous-looking machine, a hydraulic press. The press, using a high amount of pressure, squeezes out the already liquefied cocoa butter, leaving behind "cocoa cakes." The rest of the chocolate liquor moves through what look to be PVC pipes on a journey into a very big room with ceilings over forty feet tall. This is where you find the chocolate river, right? No, but it is impressive nonetheless. You may see up to six giant "bowls" in a room, with each "bowl" measuring about twenty feet high

and fifteen feet in diameter. Here you can climb up (again with the permission of a technician) and peer over the edge to see the pools of luscious, silky chocolate being mixed gently by the big metal arms. If the metal arms were not in the way, one might be tempted to swan dive into the bowl. These oversized bowls literally mix tons of sugar, milk, chocolate liquor, cocoa butter, and vanilla. Of course, the ingredients depend on the type of chocolate being made. The chocolate is now ready to be perfected. The perfection process begins with big rollers that smooth out the chocolate into different particle sizes. Here you see the chocolate being refined on a series of big metal rollers about two to three feet in diameter. They keep rolling the chocolate until the desired particle size is achieved. At this point, the wonderful chocolate aroma is pervasive, and trust us, by this point, you are strongly craving a piece of chocolate. Through the kindness of the technicians, while the big boss is not watching, you can sample the chocolate coming out of the refiner (luckily, neither one of us has ever blown up into a big blueberry from these sneaky tastings). It tastes more like chocolate at this point, but it still is not perfect. The conche will take care of that. The conching of the chocolate is a beautiful sight; several metal arms simply agitate and mix a big pool of chocolate. Once tempered, the chocolate is then transported to its final factory destination to be either molded or used to enrobe a chocolate candy bar. And finally, the best part of the experience is to see the final chocolate bars marching on the conveyor belt to be clothed (wrapped). The technicians are always kind enough to grab a couple of those little chocolate soldiers out of their line to let you taste a very fresh, newly made chocolate treat—believe us, there is nothing like it! To experience freshly made chocolate yourself, look up a local chocolate shop and find out when they first put out their newly made chocolate or you can try making chocolate yourself. (See the "Working with Chocolate" section on pp. 122–23.) We must warn you, do not be disheartened if your chocolate does not come out perfect the first time. It may take a couple of tries to refine your chocolate-making skills—at least that was our experience.

WHAT MAKES CHOCOLATE SO SPECIAL?

Aside from a rich history and its rich taste, chocolate has magnificent components. The little bean from which chocolate originates is full of Mother Nature's goodness. The ancient civilizations knew this, the Europeans quickly accepted this, and now through modern science, we can confirm this. Originating from a plant, chocolate can retain the healthy nutrients inherent in plants. The starting point, the bean, is rich in fat, carbohydrates, fiber,

Chocolate Truffle: Higher-end chocolates are typically smoother due to their smaller particle sizes achieved in the refining step.

> **Chocolate Truffle:**
> The word *conch* comes from the Spanish word *concha*, meaning shell. This term is used for chocolate because many of the original vessels that held chocolate were in the shape of a shell.

minerals, and phytonutrients (plant nutrients that can benefit our health). The end product, chocolate or cocoa powder, can retain much of this goodness, depending on the manufacturing process and the amount of cocoa solids (the nonfat, "meat" of the bean) that ends up in the finished product.

Fats

Many of us consider chocolate to be an indulgent treat that can trigger guilty feelings if we "indulge" too much. Part of this guilt is due to the fat found in chocolate. The cacao bean itself is about 50 percent fat, which is called cocoa butter but can also be called Theobroma oil (named after the tree). A typical bar of chocolate is about 30 to 45 percent fat and contains about 12 grams of fat (in a typical 40 gram or 1.3 ounce serving). Interestingly, because of the antioxidants naturally found in cocoa butter, it will not spoil or go rancid for several years. As we've seen, it is the cocoa butter that creates the luscious sensory journey that begins with the melting of chocolate on our tongues. Melting at just below body temperature, the cocoa butter begins to

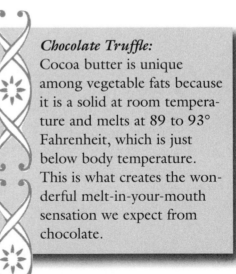

> **Chocolate Truffle:**
> Cocoa butter is unique among vegetable fats because it is a solid at room temperature and melts at 89 to 93° Fahrenheit, which is just below body temperature. This is what creates the wonderful melt-in-your-mouth sensation we expect from chocolate.

Chocolate Truffle:
The white or hazy film sometimes seen on what one might consider "old" chocolate is due to either fat- or sugar-bloom. In the case of fat-bloom, the cocoa butter was not developed properly during the manufacturing process and "leaked" out of its structure to the surface of the chocolate. This causes the chocolate to feel oily and have a dull appearance. Sugar-bloom occurs when chocolate gets humid; this can happen when refrigerated chocolate is brought into a warmer environment. The chocolate "sweats" or becomes moist, and the sugar crystals dissolve on the surface of the chocolate. When the moisture evaporates, the sugar is left on the surface and the chocolate feels grainy.

liquefy almost immediately when it touches our skin or tongue.

Cocoa butter is mainly made up of saturated fat (usually thought of as unhealthy because it often raises cholesterol levels) and monounsaturated fat (healthy fat that can lower cholesterol levels). About 36 percent of the fat in cocoa butter is monounsaturated fat and about 61 percent is saturated. Interestingly, one of the saturated fats found in cocoa butter, called stearic acid, does not increase cholesterol levels in our bodies as a typical saturated fat would. Instead, it is metabolized by our bodies into a healthy unsaturated fat. More than half of the saturated fat in cocoa butter is from stearic acid. This might explain why research shows that chocolate does not negatively impact our cholesterol levels.

Minerals

Minerals help our bodies function by participating in key reactions. Coming from the earth, cacao beans are naturally rich in minerals. As shown on p. 120, chocolate is rich in copper, iron, magnesium,

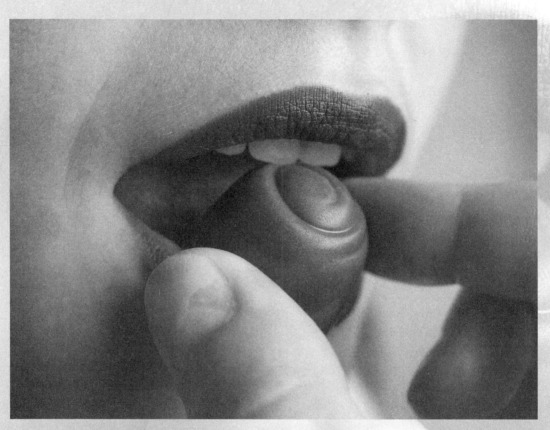

Chocolate has a perfect quality of melting just below body temperature, creating that luscious, smooth, one-of-a-kind mouth feel. Image from BigStockPhoto.com. Used with permission.

phosphorus, potassium, and zinc. In fact, finished dark chocolate and natural cocoa powders have been estimated to contribute about 9.4 percent of the daily copper intake to a typical American diet. These minerals, naturally found together in plant-based foods, work synergistically to keep us healthy. For instance, copper is believed to help maintain a healthy vascular system; potassium may decrease strokes and blood pressure; and magnesium may help maintain healthy blood sugar levels and a healthy cardiovascular system.

Chocolate Truffle:
Cocoa butter has been used to keep skin soft and supple as well as to treat skin conditions such as eczema and dermatitis for centuries. As one of the most stable, highly concentrated natural fats known, cocoa butter is readily absorbed into the skin.

MINERAL CONTENT TABLE

	Calcium (mg)	%DV	Copper (mg)	%DV	Iron (mg)	%DV	Magnesium (mg)	%DV	Phosphorus (mg)	%DV	Potassium (mg)	%DV	Zinc (mg)	%DV
Cacao Beans *Nutrient/1.5 oz*	49	5%	1.2	60%	1.5	8%	171	43%	213	21%	450	13%	1.8	12%
Cocoa Mix Powder *Nutrient/1 oz (1-envelope)*	37	4%	0.1	4%	0.3	2%	23	6%	88	9%	199	6%	0.4	3%
Milk Chocolate *Nutrient/1.4 oz*	76	8%	0.2	10%	1.0	5%	25	6%	83	8%	149	4%	0.8	5%
Semisweet Chocolate Chips *Nutrient/1 oz*	9	1%	0.2	10%	0.9	5%	33	8%	37	4%	103	3%	0.5	3%
Baking Chocolate, unsweetened *Nutrient/1 oz*	29	3%	0.9	47%	5.1	28%	95	24%	116	12%	241	7%	2.8	19%

The table shows the amounts of the minerals in the different chocolates and the percentages contributed to our daily needs, shown as %DV.

Phytonutrients

Perhaps the most exciting nutrients found in the cacao bean are the potent phytonutrients, which are credited for chocolate's resurgence into the health arena. These particular phytonutrients, called flavonoids, are the nutrients found in green tea, red wine, nuts, and many fruits. These are the same nutrients that helped make green tea and red wine appreciated in health and wellness circles. You may have also heard that blueberries have powerful antioxidants; again, this is related to their flavonoid content. Flavonoids are abundant in the beans and first piqued our interest because of their antioxidant powers. The types of flavonoids in chocolate are somewhat unique in the plant world. Unlike most plants, the bean not only has small flavonoids but is also rich in larger flavonoids. This matters because these different-sized flavonoids may provide different health benefits.

Flavonoids, similar to minerals, are found in different concentrations in our finished chocolate and cocoa products.

The amount of flavonoids contained in chocolate and cocoa are related to the type and origin of the bean; the degree of bean fermentation after harvesting (the more fermented, the lower the flavonoid content); as well as the manufacturing processes (high heat or adding alkali diminish the flavonoid content). Although these can be major factors in affecting the retention of the flavonoids, studies have shown that the flavonoid content is mostly determined by the amount of the nonfat portion of the bean, or nonfat cocoa solids, that ends up in the finished product. In other words, the general rule is, the more cocoa or higher percentage of cacao in the chocolate, the greater the flavonoid content. This is primarily because chocolate manufacturers source their beans from all over the world and often blend the beans. So many of the factors that affect flavonoid content, such as bean variety or fermentation time, do not have as great an impact. The newer chocolates of "origin"—that are made from the beans of only one region—may differ from this rule since they are not a blend and the particular bean's flavonoid content is retained. Chocolate of this kind will taste of the beans from a specific region or country as opposed to a taste blended to fit a desired taste profile.

Chocolate Truffle:
To find flavonoid-rich chocolate and cocoa, look for lightly alkalized or "Dutched" natural cocoa powder and chocolate made with at least 40 percent cacao.

WORKING WITH CHOCOLATE
(FROM WWW.GHIRARDELLI.COM WITH CULINARY INSTITUTE OF AMERICA)
Reprinted with permission of the Ghirardelli Chocolate Company.

Melting Chocolate for a Recipe

To begin, all tools and table must be completely dry. Even a couple of drops of water can make your chocolate gritty and lumpy. Also make sure not to scorch your chocolate by not going above 110 degrees. Dark chocolate can typically handle up to 120 degrees, but milk chocolate should not go above 110 degrees.

Temperature ranges:

Dark Chocolate: 114–118° F (46–48° C)
Milk Chocolate: 105–113° F (40–45° C)
White Chocolate: 100–110° F (37–43° C) Note: The high milk and sugar content in white chocolate can cause it to burn easily.

Melting Chocolate

When using a double boiler (a bowl over a pot of hot water) break your chocolate into uniform, small pieces. Using a spatula, continuously stir to help the chocolate melt. When it is almost completely melted, take it off the heat and continue to stir to help the chocolate completely melt. A candy thermometer can be used to make sure the chocolate does not get too hot.

When using a microwave, put chocolate chips or evenly chopped chocolate into a microwaveable bowl and heat on 50 percent power for one minute. Check, and if not melting, then put in for another minute. Using a dry spatula, stir and use the residual heat to finish the melting. Once you have tried stirring for about a minute to help the chocolate finish melting, you will be able to tell if you need to put it back into the microwave or not. You can also use a thermometer to check the temperature.

Tempering Chocolate

Tempering chocolate is important to create the optimal snap, sheen, and melt-in-your-mouth goodness desired in solid chocolate. By tempering the chocolate, you are actually creating the preferred type of cocoa butter crystal.

First melt your chocolate using the above instructions, again making sure everything is dry. Then you can either use the tabling or the seeding method.

Tabling

Spread melted chocolate onto a marble or granite table top—spread thin with a putty knife, continuously moving so to keep the cocoa butter uniform throughout the chocolate. Spread thin to cool quickly; as it crystallizes it will becomes firmer and firmer with a gloss. Once the chocolate holds its shape, the chocolate is tempered. Mix the tempered chocolate with the remaining melted chocolate in the bowl. The mixture should be kept at between 87 and 91 degrees.

Components of crystallized cocoa butter will allow the remaining melted cocoa butter to set very quickly. If too thick, heat up the mixture to 87–91 degrees. Above 91 degrees, the chocolate loses its shape and below 87, the chocolate will be too thick.

Seeding Method

Melt chocolate then add grated and chopped chocolate, continuously stirring until completely melted. Continue to add chocolate until the mixture is cooled to the desired temperatures below (this could take anywhere from ten to fifteen minutes).

Dark chocolate should be between 88 and 89° F (31° C).

Milk and white chocolates should be between 84 and 86° F (29 and 30° C).

Cocoa Cravings: Luscious Bites

Decadent Chocolate Truffles
Adapted by Shara Aaron and Monica Bearden

Ingredients:

Ganache (see recipe, p. 128)

Semisweet or bittersweet chocolate ranging from 60% cocoa to 70% cocoa. The chocolate should be melted and tempered. For tempering instructions, see box on pp. 122–23.

Natural cocoa powder

Cocoa nibs

Equipment:

Teaspoon
Fork
Cookie sheet
Parchment paper or aluminum foil
Plate
Small bowl

Directions:

1. Roll about ½ teaspoon of ganache into a ball between your palms. (The small balls can be irregular in shape.)

2. Place balls on a cookie sheet lined with parchment paper or a sheet of aluminum foil.

Chocolate Truffles:

1. Using a dinner fork, immerse ganache balls in melted chocolate one at a time. Make sure to completely coat with chocolate.

2. If you have tempered your own chocolate, make sure to cool to 70° F (or below) at room temperature or by using the refrigerator.

3. If you are using untempered chocolate, place in the refrigerator and keep cool until ready to eat.

Chocolate Truffles with Cocoa Powder
(see the color insert photo of cocoa truffles):

1. Spread natural cocoa powder in a thin layer on a plate or cookie sheet.

2. Completely coat the ganache balls with the powder by gently rolling.

Chocolate Truffles with Cocoa Nibs
(the meat of the cacao bean
left after roasting and winnowing):

1. Sprinkle a few tablespoons of cocoa nibs in a small bowl.

2. Completely coat the ganache with the nibs by gently rolling.

3. Ganache is an emulsion of chocolate and cream. Use either semisweet or bittersweet chocolate, ranging from 60% to 70% cocoa.

Chocolate Ganache

Ingredients:

6 ounces semisweet or bittersweet chocolate, finely
chopped
½ to ¾ cup heavy cream

Equipment:

Mixing bowl
Rubber spatula
Small saucepan
2- or 3-quart double boiler or
mixing bowl and
saucepan
Candy thermometer

Directions:

1. Melt the chocolate until it reaches a temperature of about 120° F in a bowl over a pot of simmering water or in the top of a double boiler.

2. Bring the cream to a boil in a small saucepan then remove from heat and cool in a stainless steel bowl.

3. When the cream has cooled to about 115° F, slowly pour the chocolate into the cream (the temperature of the chocolate should not be lower than 110° F; if so, briefly reheat it to 115° F).

4. As you pour, stir with the rubber spatula, thoroughly mixing the chocolate into the cream. The mixture will thicken and should be smooth and shiny.

5. Cool to room temperature. If cooling in a refrigerator to room temperature, cover with plastic wrap.

6. Once cooled the consistency of the ganache best suited for making truffles is that of peanut butter or slightly stiffer.

Dark Chocolate Nut Clusters

by Tina Casey (compliments of www.Chocoholic.com—
your connection to the world of Premium Chocolates)

Directions:

1. Prepare one or two large cookie sheets by lining them with lightly greased waxed paper.

2. Place dark chocolate in a lightly greased crock pot set to low (if you don't have a crock pot, you can use a heavy pan on the lowest setting of the stove . . . but you must watch the chocolate carefully, as it will melt more quickly and at a higher temperature. Or use a double boiler, but be sure to simmer very gently and check the water level).

3. Allow it to melt very slowly, for about two, or even three-plus hours, stirring occasionally.

4. When chocolate is completely melted, add nuts and stir, making sure to thoroughly coat nuts.

5. Drop by tablespoon onto wax-papered cookie sheets and let cool and harden in a cool place, for several hours or overnight.

Store in tight jars or tins.

Ingredients:

24 ounces of solid, bittersweet dark chocolate
1 pound of fresh, dry-roasted,
  or unsalted almonds or
  peanuts
Crock pot or heavy deep pan
One or two large cookie
  sheets, lined with lightly
  greased wax paper

Molded Chocolate Turtles
Traditional recipe adapted by Shara Aaron and Monica Bearden

Ingredients:

Caramel Filling:

13.5 ounces white chocolate,
    chopped
½ cup granulated sugar
3 tablespoons water
1 cup heavy cream, warmed
¼ teaspoon salt
2 tablespoons unsalted butter,
    cut into tablespoons

Candied Pecans:

2 cups whole pecans
¼ cup light corn syrup

Chocolate Coating:
15 ounces dark chocolate,
    coarsely chopped

Directions:

Caramel filling:

1. Place white chocolate in medium bowl and set aside.

2. Place sugar and water in heavy-bottomed saucepan and cook over medium heat, stirring until sugar dissolves. Stop stirring and increase heat to high.

3. Cook, occasionally brushing down sides of pan with wet pastry brush, until mixture turns dark golden brown.

4. Slowly and carefully add warm heavy cream and salt and mix until combined and smooth.

5. Pour hot mixture over chopped chocolate and let stand for a minute to allow chocolate to melt.

6. Stir until combined; add butter and mix until smooth.

7. Cool to room temperature.

Candied pecans:

1. Preheat oven to 325° F.
2. Place pecans in medium bowl.
3. Place corn syrup in heavy-bottomed saucepan over medium-high heat and cook until very warm.
4. Pour over pecans and toss until pecans are fully coated.
5. Place on a parchment paper– or foil-lined baking sheet and bake for 15 minutes.
6. Place baking sheet on wire rack and cool completely.

Assembly:

1. Place wire rack over foil-lined baking sheet.
2. Place chocolate in microwave-able bowl.
3. Microwave on medium (50% power) for 1½ minutes.
4. Stir. Continue microwaving and stirring in 1 ½-minute intervals until chocolate is melted and smooth.
5. Fill tablet molds with chocolate, then turn them upside down onto rack to allow excess to drip out.
6. After a few minutes, when chocolate just begins to set, scrape edges of cavities with dull side of chef's knife to make a clean edge.
7. When chocolate has completely set, fill with caramel filling to about ⅛ inch from top, spreading it evenly with a small spatula.
8. Place in refrigerator for about 20 minutes.
9. Remove from refrigerator.
10. Cover filling with a thin layer of melted chocolate to seal. Let set at room temperature for 5 minutes.
11. Sprinkle chocolate with a few candied pecans, pressing them very lightly onto the chocolate.
12. Return to refrigerator for another 30 minutes or until set.
13. Remove from refrigerator. Invert gently to release tablets from molds.

Chapter 4

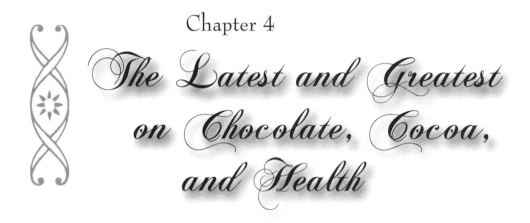

The Latest and Greatest on Chocolate, Cocoa, and Health

"I don't understand why so many 'so-called' chocolate lovers complain about the calories in chocolate, when all true chocoholics know that it is a vegetable. It comes from the cacao bean, beans are veggies, 'nuff said."

Unknown

"There are four basic food groups: milk chocolate, dark chocolate, white chocolate, and chocolate truffles."

Anonymous

"I have this theory that chocolate slows down the aging process. . . . It may not

be true, but do I dare take the chance?"

Unknown

Throughout history cocoa and chocolate were beloved for their health-giving properties, but for much of the twentieth century, chocolate was demonized as a high-fat, high-calorie food, offering no more than pleasure. All of that changed about a decade ago when the first news reports came out that cocoa contains plant compounds that may be good for you. On

133

February 14, 2002, a *New York Times* headline read: "Valentine to Dark Chocolate, but Go Easy." Many of the first reports gave caveats that chocolate "might possibly have something in it that can benefit health," but to be careful about eating it too often since it's high in calories and fat. Other news reports were highly skeptical and bashed the whole notion of chocolate having health benefits. However, we've come a long way since then and have come to understand that cocoa and chocolate (in moderation) can be enjoyed each day without adverse effects for most people. The introduction of new products that have a high cocoa content (the healthy part of chocolate) can achieve health benefits in relatively small portions.

And even more exciting is the development of cocoa-based products that provide that beloved chocolate flavor and nutrient-rich cocoa but with less fat and typically fewer calories than a chocolate bar.

We, the authors, were fortunate enough to play an integral part in the early research studies in the lab but also spent years informing the public of these exciting new results. We even got to contribute to the development of new chocolate products made to benefit cardiovascular health. The boom in dark and semisweet chocolates over the past seven years is a result of the media frenzy from the science we're about to share with you. The story begins by looking through a microscope to discover the fascinating group of flavonoid compounds called flavanols.

CHOCOLATE AND COCOA: PLANT-BASED FOOD

Cocoa flavanols were discovered almost by accident. For years, manufacturers took most of the flavanols out because they imparted bitter flavor to the finished cocoa or chocolate product. Flavanols attracted interest from chocolate companies when their scientists discovered that the compounds were similar to those in tea, which had already been shown to provide health benefits.

So what exactly are these flavanols and why are they in cocoa to begin with?

Plants naturally contain compounds called phytonutrients, which protect them from environmental stresses such as ultraviolet light or pests. Phytonutrients are a relatively new category of nutrient and they do not necessarily cause a deficiency disease when the diet is lacking in them (such as anemia with iron deficiency). However, we are coming to understand that these compounds seem to have protective effects for humans by guarding against diseases, such as heart disease and cancer. So perhaps a traditional deficiency does not appear when the diet lacks a type of phytonutrient, but long-term, chronic diseases may be the result. Research is looking into these very questions.

Cacao beans, being of plant origin, are particularly rich in the phytonutrients called flavanols. Without going into too much chemistry, flavanols are molecules

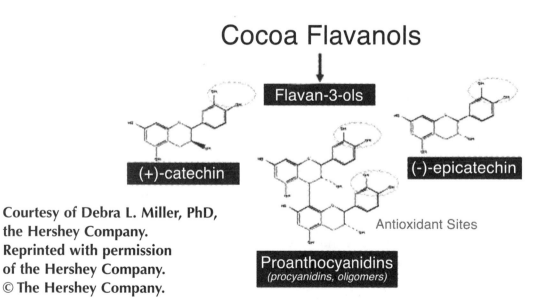

Cocoa Flavanols

Flavan-3-ols

(+)-catechin

(-)-epicatechin

Proanthocyanidins
(procyanidins, oligomers)

Antioxidant Sites

Courtesy of Debra L. Miller, PhD, the Hershey Company. Reprinted with permission of the Hershey Company. © The Hershey Company.

with a ring shape that can be single units or linked together to form long chains. Cocoa is believed to be special because it contains both smaller and larger flavanols. The structure of the different flavanol molecules plays an important part in flavanol's action as an antioxidant (a substance that protects the body's cells from the damaging effects of oxidation), which is one of the reasons that flavanols may protect against the development of diseases.

CHOCOLATE AND BLUEBERRIES: WHAT THEY HAVE IN COMMON

Blueberries—along with many other fruits, vegetables, *and cocoa*—have a healthy reputation thanks to their high quantity of antioxidants. It is these antioxidants that are credited for the health benefits of berries as well as other fruits and vegetables. A test called ORAC (oxygen radical absorbance capacity) compares the ability of foods and beverages to stop free radicals: in other words, it rates the strength or power of the antioxidants. By ranking foods according to their antioxidant power, you can choose the foods that may have stronger free radical protection. Chocolate and cocoa are naturally rich in antioxidants and when ranked with other antioxidant-packed foods, like blueberries, they can have as much as two to three times the antioxidant power of other plant-based foods!

YOUR VASCULAR SYSTEM LOVES CHOCOLATE TOO!

Healthy blood flow is a vital aspect of overall health because blood carries all of the nutrients and oxygen that are needed

> *Chocolate Truffle:*
> More than 10 percent of the weight of the dry raw cacao beans consists of phytonutrients alone. (allchocolate.com)

What Are Antioxidants?

Antioxidant is a term that is thrown around in today's vernacular often with little understanding of what it really means. Whenever we ask someone what is an antioxidant, the most common answer is "I don't know, but it's good for you." Here's the definition:

An antioxidant is any molecule capable of slowing or preventing another molecule from becoming oxidized. It's bad when other molecules are oxidized because it means they are highly charged and can damage the nearby cells as they roam the body. These free radicals or charged molecules may be neutralized when they come in contact with an antioxidant. It is similar to billiards; the cue stick hits the cue ball, giving it a lot of energy, and thus creating the free radical. The cue ball, which is out of control, in turn, bumps and hits the other balls, knocking them into the pockets or sides of the table (disrupting them from their resting state). An antioxidant would stop the cue ball from moving around uncontrollably and would keep it from disturbing the other balls.

throughout the body. Many of the benefits of flavanols are due to their protective effects on the blood vessels. By keeping the blood vessels healthy, blood flow can be more efficient, which is beneficial for all of your organs. To function properly, all biological systems—including the cardio-vascular system, kidneys, eyes, brain, skin, and muscles—rely on a healthy supply of blood.

One way that flavanols help to keep our vessels healthy is by keeping platelets from getting sticky. Platelets are blood

Chocolate Truffle:
According to the USDA, two tablespoons of natural cocoa have more antioxidant capacity than four cups of green tea, one cup of blue-berries, or one and half glasses of red wine.

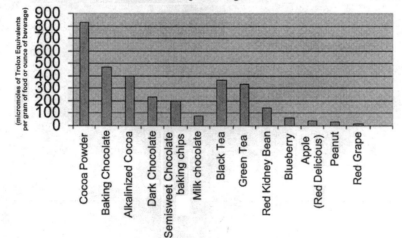

Total Antioxidant Capacity of foods as measured

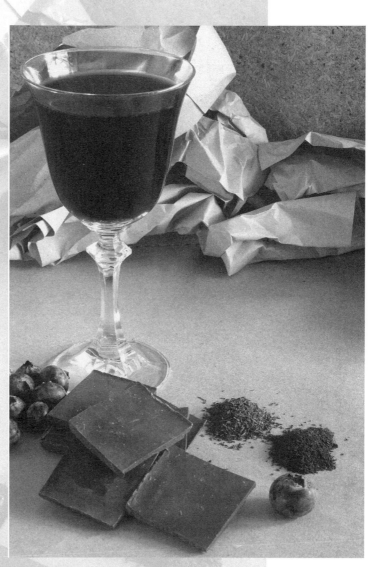

Natural cocoa and dark chocolate have more antioxidant power than blueberries or red wine.
© Sandra Caldwell. Image from BigStockPhoto.com. Used with permission.

How Many Flavanols Do You Need?

Although there is no official recommended daily amount of flavanols, as there is for calcium and fiber, researchers do have a good understanding of what is an effective dose. Studies show beneficial effects on blood vessels, blood pressure, and inflammation with intakes as low as 150–200 mg of flavanols per day. As the amount of flavanols increases, the health benefits are even more pronounced. The current estimated average intake of flavanols in the United States is 58 mg per day.

Flavanol Content in Foods

Food, serving size	Flavanols
Cranberries, 1 cup	419 mg
Blueberries, 1 cup	266 mg
Apple, 1 medium	229 mg
Strawberries, 1 cup halves	220 mg
Hazelnuts, 1 oz.	143 mg
Grape juice, 1 cup	124 mg
Red wine, 5 oz.	91 mg
Almonds, 1 oz.	53 mg
Black tea, 6 oz.	24 mg

Source: Prior et al., J Agric. Food Chem. 2004

Flavanol Content of Chocolates and Cocoas

Food, standard serving size	Flavanols/ standard serving
Dark chocolate, 40 g (1.4 oz.)	517 mg
Unsweetened baking chocolate, 15 g (1 Tbs.)	312 mg
Natural cocoa powder, 5 g (1 Tbs.)	204 mg
Semisweet baking chips, 15 g (1 Tbs.)	184 mg
Milk chocolate, 40 g (1.4 oz.)	108 mg
Dutched cocoa powder, 5 g (1 Tbs.)	45 mg

Source: Gu et al. 2006

cells that can block blood flow if they clump together. Flavanols reduce the tendency for platelets to stick together. In studies published in the *American Journal of Clinical Nutrition* in 2000 and *Thrombosis Research* in 2002, participants consumed flavanol-rich chocolate or a flavanol-rich cocoa beverage, and researchers saw reduced platelet activity, similar to the reduced clotting action of a baby aspirin. Again, flavanols help to keep blood flowing smoothly.

Research also shows that flavanols may decrease inflammation. Inflammation is the body's immune response to infection or a foreign substance. Your body contains both anti- and pro-inflammatory compounds. Each is a necessary part of the immune response. The anti-inflammatories stop the immune response to injury once the body has healed, and the pro-inflammatories turn on the response when the body needs to heal. In response to an injury, such as a cut, inflammation triggers an appropriate reaction from the immune system. If the inflammation continues for too long or gets out of control, however, it can be dangerous to your health. For example, when bad cholesterol gets embedded in artery walls, the immune system sees it as an invader to be attacked and calls in the pro-inflammatories. If the inflammation continues for a long period of time, it can cause a revved-up immune response and lead to a buildup of plaque. It is the bursting or movement of the enlarged plaque that can then cause a heart attack or stroke. The ongoing inflammation in arteries can create a revved-up immune response. This can further damage arteries and cause plaque to build up and even burst, causing a heart attack or stroke. Chronic inflammation appears to play a role in such medical evils, from arthritis to Alzheimer's to diabetes to heart disease. By improving the ratio of anti-inflammatory compounds to pro-inflammatory compounds, flavanols decrease inflammation. And by reducing inflammation, flavanol-rich cocoa and chocolate may in turn decrease the incidence of multiple diseases.

Additionally, flavanols may improve blood flow and vascular health by helping blood vessels widen or dilate.

Blood pressure has been shown to be lowered by eating flavanol-rich cocoa and chocolate. In studies people who ate a small daily dosage of cocoa (4.2 grams/day or 10 grams/day of dark chocolate) experienced a lowered systolic and diastolic blood pressure (both parts of the blood pressure reading you receive from your doctor). They also had a lower risk of heart disease and death from all causes. These studies suggest that long-term daily intake of a small amount of cocoa may lower blood pressure and offer disease protection.

Another ongoing study from Harvard University looked at the rate of high blood pressure in the Kuna population—a group of people with traditionally low rates of hypertension and cardiovascular disease. Researchers compared the Kuna living a more traditional lifestyle on an island off the coast of Panama with those who had migrated to the city on the mainland and consumed a more Westernized diet. Researchers found that the traditional diet contained about four eight-ounce cups of a cocoa beverage high in flavanols as well as abundant amounts of fruit and fish. They also noted that both groups consumed high amounts of salt. Only those Kuna following the traditional diet—rich in flavanols—experienced low rates of hypertension.

CHOCOLATE AND YOUR IMMUNE SYSTEM

The immune system provides wonderful and necessary actions in a healthy body to fight off invaders such as bacteria and viruses; however, when the system goes awry and kicks into overdrive, numerous health conditions arise. Similar to cocoa's ability to reduce inflammation, the flavanols that are naturally found in chocolate have been shown to directly affect the immune system: they suppress compounds that create harmful immune responses in the body. As noted earlier, this can be helpful in controlling overly active immune responses that are responsible for arthritis, heart disease, and autoimmune diseases.

EAT CHOCOLATE TO STAY SHARP: THE COGNITIVE BENEFITS OF COCOA

Always forgetting where you put your keys? You may need a daily dose of cocoa. Thanks to its ability to promote blood flow, cocoa may enhance brain function, as several new studies have indicated. In one study at the University of Nottingham in 2006, sixteen people consumed a high-flavanol cocoa drink (150 mg of cocoa flavanols) for five days and then performed two reactive tasks, including pressing a button when seeing certain letters and numbers. The researchers measured reaction time and error rate as well as changes in blood flow to the brain. They then repeated the experiment after participants consumed a low-flavanol drink. The activity in the neurons (which are the message wires in the brain) and changes in blood flow in the brain increased when participants drank the high-flavanol cocoa but had no change with the low-flavanol drink. The flavanol-rich cocoa had no effect, nonetheless, on behavior such as reaction time or error rate during the tasks. Still, the researchers contend that the blood flow changes and activity in the brain rather than behavioral changes are a better indicator of underlying brain function. A prior study at the same lab at the University of Nottingham involving four subjects with just a single high dose (450 mg flavanols) of flavanol-rich cocoa also showed an increase in blood flow in the brain. The researchers concluded that "the increase in blood flow to key areas of the brain could indicate a potential use for cocoa flavanols in the treatment of vascular impairment, including dementia and stroke."

At Harvard University another study in 2006 involved the daily ingestion of 900 mg of flavanols for one week. It showed an increase in blood flow to the brain in healthy elderly subjects. A decrease in brain blood flow has been seen in patients with dementia and is associated with cognitive decline. By improving vascular blood flow to the brain, cocoa flavanols may have some potential for reducing the risk of dementia, although much more research is needed in this area.

THE BEAUTY BENEFITS OF CHOCOLATE

Cocoa butter has long been used as a topical beauty product because of its moisturizing properties. Interestingly, drinking or eating cocoa and chocolate may help improve the look of skin as well. It is not necessarily, however, due to the cocoa butter but is related to the cocoa flavanols, their antioxidant actions and ability to increase blood flow to the skin. In a novel study at the University of Dusseldorf in 2006, two groups of women consumed a high-flavanol (326 mg) or low-flavanol (26 mg) cocoa drink each day for twelve weeks. Researchers exposed selected skin areas to solar-simulated radiation. After measuring the redness of the skin from the UV exposure, they looked at peripheral blood flow and hydration in the skin. They saw reductions in skin redness in the high-flavanol group and no change in the low-flavanol group. The positive results included an increase in blood flow as well as an increase in density and thickness of the skin. There was also a decrease in water loss from the skin, thus helping the

Chocolate Truffle:
A compound called phenylethylamine (PEA) may be responsible for some of the pleasurable feelings you experience after eating chocolate, since it releases natural feel-good chemicals called endorphins in your brain. PEA is released by the brain when people are falling in love.

skin to stay more moisturized naturally. The cocoa flavanols protected the skin from UV damage, improved blood circulation to the skin, maintained skin hydration, and improved overall appearance of the skin.

Another study published in the *European Journal of Nutrition* in 2007 found that peripheral blood flow to the skin increased after drinking a high-flavanol cocoa drink with no change after consumption of a low-flavanol cocoa drink. The observed effect is likely due to the ability of cocoa flavanols to dilate blood vessels and improve blood flow. So using cocoa both externally and internally can improve the look and health of skin.

CHOCOLATE AND BLOOD SUGAR

Most people think that cocoa and chocolate are bad news for blood sugar control. Chocolate is blamed for sugar spikes and crashes among the young and not-so-young. Those afflicted with diabetes (a disease related to the body's ability to control high blood sugar) especially believe that chocolate is on the no-no list. New research is enlightening us every day. In fact, according to new research, fitting chocolate into a healthful diet may possibly offer some health benefits in regard to blood sugar control. High blood sugar can negatively affect circulation and blood vessels. Because flavanols have the ability to improve blood flow and keep vessels healthy, a diet rich in flavanols may possibly benefit those concerned with blood sugar control.

Another emerging area of study is cocoa's and chocolate's impact on insulin sensitivity, a crucial issue for those concerned with maintaining healthy blood sugar levels. Insulin is the hormone in the body that takes sugar out of the blood and helps it into the cells, where it is needed for energy. With a decreased sensitivity to insulin, cells cannot pull sugar out of the bloodstream for their use. This creates elevated levels of blood sugar, and can result in diabetes or hyperglycemia. In a small study from the *American Journal of Clinical Nutrition* in 2004, researchers found that when flavanol-rich chocolate was given to participants for fifteen days, blood sugar levels became lower than before the treatment period. This suggests that flavanol-rich chocolate may possibly help to increase insulin sensitivity, thus it might possibly help to control blood sugar levels. Nevertheless, the research is preliminary. More research with larger numbers of participants is needed to confirm and understand chocolate's potential effect on the prevention and treatment of diabetes. For now, those with diabetes should consult their doctors regarding their diets and can work with a dietitian to include cocoa or high-cocoa-content chocolates in their diet.

OTHER RESEARCH FINDINGS OF INTEREST

There is scientific evidence to indicate that cocoa, chocolate, and the flavanols they contain inhibit numerous diseases. By improving blood flow, keeping vessels healthy, and acting as an antioxidant, flavanols affect many systems within the body. Thus far, the research has looked at measurements that are linked to diseases.

Chocolate Truffle:
Despite its sweet reputation, dark chocolate has a low glycemic index (a measure of how foods impact blood sugar) similar to that of oatmeal—meaning it does not necessarily send your blood sugar spiking.

For example, elevated blood pressure increases risk of heart disease; cocoa flavanols can lower blood pressure and could potentially impact heart disease risk. One of the more challenging diseases to study is cancer. The disease is quite complex and many mechanisms contribute to its development. New studies are researching flavanols' potential anticancer effects. A study at Georgetown University in 2005 noted that breast cancer cells have been shown to stop multiplying when combined with specific flavanols in a test tube. Similar results have been seen on prostate cancer cells in a study published in the *European Journal of Cancer Prevention* in 2006. These studies are promising, but researchers are only at the very beginning of understanding the potential anticancer effects of cocoa flavanols.

HOW TO CHOOSE YOUR CHOCOLATES FOR FLAVANOL CONTENT

As we've seen, flavanols are an important nutrient in chocolate and cocoa and pro-

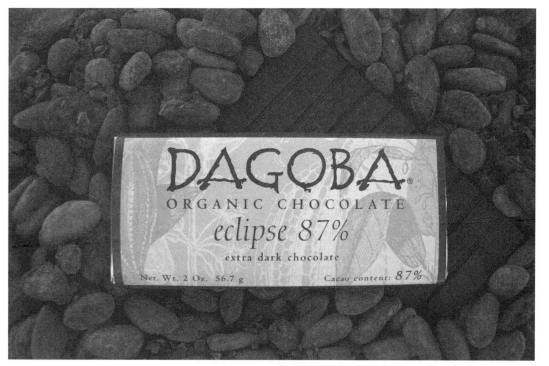

More and more chocolates have their %cacao listed on the label. Choosing higher %cacao chocolates typically means more flavanols. Reprinted with permission of Artisan Confections Company. © Artisan Confections Company.

vide a bounty of health benefits. Unfortunately, flavanols are not a nutrient typically found on a food label. So how do you know what to look for when choosing a chocolate for its flavanol content? Studies have found that while the processing of cocoa in the chocolate can affect its flavanol content—non- or lightly alkalized retain flavanols better than alkalized—the most essential component in determining the flavanol content is the total amount of nonfat cocoa solids, or as it will say on the package, % cacao (or % cocoa). The bottom line: in most cases, the higher the % cacao (or % cocoa), the greater the amount of flavanols in the product.

Some companies, especially the large ones, such as Mars, Incorporated and the Hershey Company, have tested many of their products with the US Department of Agriculture to determine their flavanol content. They may even print the number of flavanols on the packaging or at least have it available if you call their consumer affairs departments. More often than not, however, you won't know the exact number of flavanols in your chocolate, so you may want to refer to the chart "Flavanol Content of Chocolates and Cocoas" on p. 140 for a general guideline.

Because you or a loved one chose this book, you are clearly a lover of chocolate. Your first and foremost infatuation likely derived from the delicious, heartwarming taste that chocolate offers. But as you can see, cocoa, chocolate, and nature's gift of flavanols to these foods, provide numerous health benefits that are not only real but are supported by science. Armed with this new information, you may find yourself with a new appreciation and perspective when passing by a heart-shaped box full of chocolates.

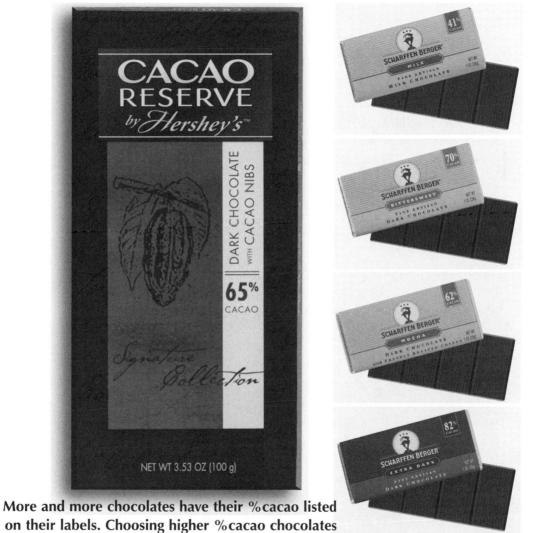

More and more chocolates have their %cacao listed on their labels. Choosing higher %cacao chocolates typically means more flavanols.
Reprinted with permission of the Hershey Company.
© The Hershey Company.

The Chocolate Manufacturers Association Provides Tips for Healthy Ways of Eating Cocoa and Chocolate.

- Sprinkle cocoa powder on popcorn, warm and cold coffee drinks, low-fat or nonfat plain yogurt mixed with fresh fruit, and baked pears, apples, or other fruit.
- Mix small bite-size pieces of dark chocolate in with a homemade trail mix of nuts and dried fruits.
- Add chocolate shavings or cocoa nibs to fresh fruit cups, salad greens, or cold cereals such as granola or warm cereals such as oatmeal or cream of wheat.
- Dip fresh or dried fruits such as strawberries, bananas, or dried apricots into chocolate.
- Add semisweet chocolate chips into easy-to-bake vegetable breads or cakes such as banana bread, pumpkin bread, or carrot cake.
- Incorporate into sauces such as Mexican molé.

Cocoa Cravings: Healthy Recipes

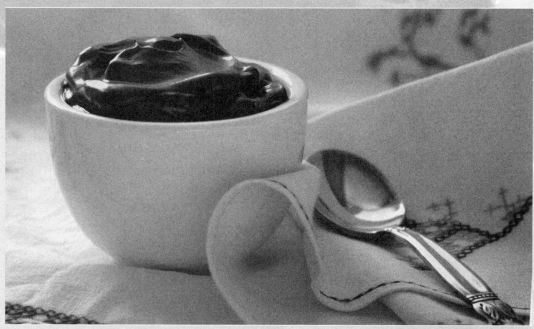

© Alice Day.
Image from BigStockPhoto.com.
Used with permission.

Lighter-Than-Air Chocolate Delight

Recipe courtesy of the Hershey Kitchens and reprinted with permission of the Hershey Company. © The Hershey Company.

Ingredients:

2 envelopes unflavored gelatin

½ cup cold water

1 cup boiling water

1⅓ cups nonfat dry milk powder

⅓ cup Hershey's Special Dark Cocoa or Hershey's Cocoa

1 tablespoon vanilla extract

Dash of salt

Granulated sugar substitute to equal 14 teaspoons sugar

8 large ice cubes

Directions:

1. Sprinkle gelatin over cold water in blender container; let stand 4 minutes to soften.

2. Gently stir with rubber spatula, scraping gelatin particles off sides; add boiling water to gelatin mixture.

3. Cover; blend until gelatin dissolves.

4. Add dry milk powder, cocoa, vanilla, and salt; blend on medium speed until well mixed.

5. Add sugar substitute and ice cubes; blend on high speed until ice is crushed and mixture is smooth and fluffy.

6. Immediately pour into 4-cup mold. Cover; refrigerate until firm. Unmold onto serving plate. 8 servings.

NOTE: Eight individual dessert dishes may be used in place of 4-cup mold, if desired.

Lower-Fat Iced Cappuccino

Recipe courtesy of the Hershey Kitchens and reprinted with permission of the Hershey Company. © The Hershey Company.

Ingredients:

⅔ cup Hershey's Syrup, chilled
2 cups cold coffee
2 cups lowfat vanilla ice
    cream or frozen yogurt
Ice cubes or crushed ice
Fat-free whipped topping
    (optional)
Ground cinnamon (optional)

Directions:

1. Place syrup and coffee in blender container; cover and blend on high speed.

2. Add ice cream; cover and blend until smooth.

3. Serve immediately over ice; top with whipped topping and ground cinnamon, if desired.

Makes six 6-ounce servings.

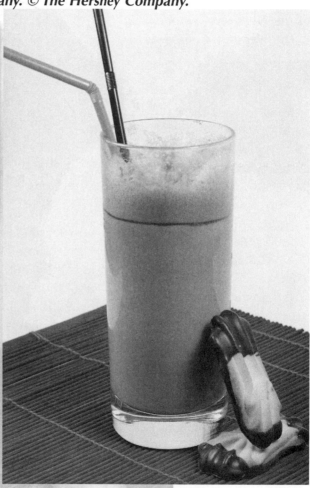

© Anna Karwowska. Image from
BigStockPhoto.com. Used with permission.

Bouquet of Pancakes

Recipe courtesy of the Hershey Kitchens and reprinted with permission of the Hershey Company.
© The Hershey Company.

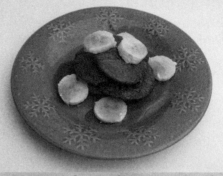

© **Martha Buchanan. Image from BigStockPhoto.com. Used with permission.**

Ingredients:

1½ cups all-purpose flour
⅔ cup sugar
½ cup Hershey's Cocoa
1 teaspoon baking powder
1 teaspoon baking soda
2 cups buttermilk
2 eggs, beaten
¼ cup plus 2 tablespoons vegetable oil
"Flowers" made from selection of sliced strawberries, sliced almonds, mandarin orange segments, sliced kiwi fruit, pineapple chunks, and maraschino cherry halves
Frozen whipped topping, thawed

Directions:

1. Stir together flour, sugar, cocoa, baking powder, and baking soda in large bowl.

2. Combine buttermilk, eggs, and oil in separate bowl; add all at once to flour mixture. Stir just until moistened.

3. Pour about 1 tablespoon batter onto preheated, lightly greased griddle or nonstick skillet. Cook over medium heat until surface bubbly on top; turn and cook until set.

4. Serve each pancake topped with heaping teaspoonful of whipped topping, topped with selection of fruits as flowers. About 40 small pancakes.

NOTE: Leftover pancakes may be tightly wrapped and frozen for later use. To reheat: Place 5 pancakes on microwave-safe plate in circular pattern; cover with wax paper. Microwave at high for 1 minute or until warm.

Citrus-Infused Bittersweet Chocolate Sauce

Recipe courtesy of www.allchocolate.com and reprinted with permission of the Hershey Company. © The Hershey Company.

Chocolate and citrus are a delectable combination. Pour this light, tangy sauce over pound cake, cheesecake, or any other dessert that needs a sweet topping!

Ingredients:

4 ounces bittersweet chocolate, broken into pieces
¼ cup light corn syrup
2 tablespoons butter or margarine
¼ cup milk
½ teaspoon vanilla extract
¼ teaspoon freshly grated orange peel

Directions:

1. Combine chocolate, corn syrup, and butter in small saucepan.
2. Cook over medium heat, stirring constantly, until chocolate is melted and mixture is smooth.
3. Gradually add milk, stirring and cooking until smooth.
4. Remove from heat.
5. Stir in vanilla and orange peel. Cool slightly.
6. Serve warm or cool over ice cream or other desserts. Cover; refrigerate leftover sauce.

Makes about 1 cup sauce

Chocolate-Dipped Dried Plums
Courtesy of the California Dried Plum Board

Ingredients:

1 cup (about 6 ounces)
   pitted dried plums
6 ounces semisweet
   chocolate, coarsely
   chopped

Fillings:

Nuts
Candied ginger
Prepared almond paste
   or marzipan

Toppings:

Chopped nuts
Candied ginger pieces
Candy decorations

Directions:

1. Cut slit into side of each dried plum; stuff with small piece or portion of filling, as desired.

2. Pinch to close; shape to form round shape. Set aside.

3. Place chocolate in small heatproof bowl, set in pot of hot (not boiling) water over low heat; allow to melt, stirring occasionally until smooth. (Chocolate should be fluid and barely warm.)

4. Remove from heat.

5. Line baking sheet with aluminum foil or wax paper.

6. Using a fork, dip dried plums, one at a time, into chocolate; drain excess. Place on prepared baking sheet and decorate with toppings as desired.

7. Refrigerate immediately until set. When chocolate has hardened, transfer to jars or containers for gift-giving.

8. Store, covered, in cool place, away from direct sun or heat.

Tip: Melted white chocolate can be drizzled over chocolate-dipped dried plums instead of or before adding toppings, if desired.

Yield: 12 servings—2 each

Cocoa Angel Food Cake
Courtesy of Chocolate Manufacturers Association (www.chocolateusa.org)

Cocoa adds an extra flavor dimension to a classic angel food cake. Serve this accompanied with a scoop of chocolate ice cream, chocolate sorbet, or drizzled with hot fudge sauce. Fresh fruit is also a good accompaniment. The cake travels well, too, so pack some slices in with your next picnic.

Ingredients:

1 cup sifted flour
3 tablespoons unsweet-
ened natural cocoa
powder, sifted
¼ teaspoon salt
1½ cups superfine sugar
12 large egg whites, at
room temperature
1 teaspoon cream of tartar
1 tablespoon pure vanilla
extract

Directions:

1. Position a rack in the center of the oven and preheat the oven to 325° F.

2. In a 1-quart bowl, thoroughly blend the flour with the cocoa powder, salt, and ¾ cup of the superfine sugar. Set this mixture aside. Place the remaining ¾ cup superfine sugar in a measuring cup near the mixer.

3. In the grease-free bowl of an electric stand mixer using the wire whip or in a mixing bowl using a handheld mixer, whip the egg whites on low speed until they are slightly frothy.

4. Add the cream of tartar and whip the egg whites until they begin to mound. While the egg whites are whipping on medium speed, slowly sprinkle on the remaining ¾ cup of superfine sugar, 2 tablespoons at a time. Then continue

whipping the whites until they are firm, but not dry.

5. Blend in the vanilla, then remove the bowl from the mixer.

6. Sprinkle the dry ingredients over the whipped egg whites, 3 tablespoons at a time and gently fold them into the whites, using a long-handled rubber spatula.

7. Turn the batter into a 10 × 4-inch tube pan, preferably with a removable bottom. Use the rubber spatula to smooth and even the top. Tap the pan on the countertop gently a few times to eliminate any air bubbles.

8. Bake the cake in the preheated oven until it is golden brown, springs back when lightly touched, and a cake tester inserted near the center comes out clean (about 40 minutes). Remove the pan from the oven and immediately invert it onto its feet, or hang it by the center tube over a funnel or the neck of a bottle. Leave the cake to hang for several hours, until it is completely cool.

9. To remove the cake from the pan, run a thin-bladed knife around the inside of the pan and around the tube. Gently loosen the cake from the edges and push the bottom of the pan up, away from the sides. Run the knife between the bottom of the cake and the bottom of the pan and invert the cake onto a plate, then reinvert, so it is right side up. Angel food cake is best cut with a serrated knife using a sawing motion.

10. The cake will keep at room temperature, well wrapped in plastic, for 3 days, or it can be frozen for up to 3 weeks. If frozen, defrost in the refrigerator for 24 hours before serving.

Makes one 10 × 3½-inch cake,
14 to 16 servings

Chocolate Sorbet
Courtesy of Chocolate Manufacturers Association (www.chocolateusa.org)

This is a smooth and intensely chocolate sorbet that is excellent on its own, but superb with chocolate pound cake, cocoa angel food cake (see recipe on p. 157), biscotti, or fresh fruit.

Directions:

1. Combine the water and sugar in a 2-quart saucepan and bring to a boil over medium heat to dissolve the sugar.

2. Add the cocoa powder and stir until it is dissolved and smooth. Remove the pan from the heat and add the chopped chocolate. Stir until it is completely melted.

3. Strain the mixture into a bowl. Cover tightly with plastic wrap and cool to room temperature. Chill for several hours or overnight, then process in an ice cream maker according to the manufacturer's instructions.

Yield: 1 pint

Ingredients:

1 ¼ cups water
¾ cup superfine sugar
⅓ cup unsweetened
   Dutch-processed
   cocoa powder, sifted
4 ounces bittersweet or
   semisweet chocolate,
   finely chopped

Chocolate-Covered Strawberries

Recipe courtesy of the Hershey Kitchens and reprinted with permission of the Hershey Company. © The Hershey Company.

Ingredients:

2 cups (12-oz. pkg.) Hershey's Special Dark Chocolate Chips or Hershey's Semisweet Chocolate Chips
2 tablespoons trans fat–free shortening (do not use butter, margarine, spread, or oil)*
Fresh strawberries, with stems, rinsed and patted dry

*Butter, margarine, and spreads contain water, which may prevent chocolate from melting properly; oil may prevent chocolate from forming a coating.

Directions:

1. Cover tray with wax paper.
2. Place chocolate chips and shortening in medium microwave-safe bowl. Microwave at medium (50% power) 1½ minutes or just until chips are melted and mixture is smooth when stirred; cool slightly.
3. Holding strawberry by top, dip ⅔ of each berry into chocolate mixture; shake gently to remove excess. Place on prepared tray.
4. Refrigerate until coating is firm, about 30 minutes. Store, covered, in refrigerator. Coats about 5 dozen small strawberries (about 1 cup coating).

Variations:

Chocolate-dipped biscotti, chocolate-covered figs, chocolate-covered dried apricots.

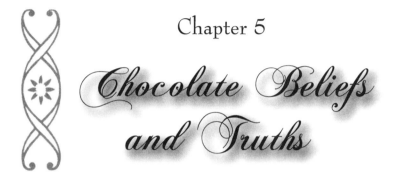

Chapter 5

Chocolate Beliefs and Truths

Many myths cloud the truth about chocolate to this day. Physicians, parents, and people in general have based medical treatments and their beliefs regarding nutrition on cause and effect. Today, health practitioners, families, and individuals all seem to have their own set of beliefs and sometimes interpret science and the news in their own personal way. Picture a mother giving her son a chocolate treat and the child jumping for joy and running around. It is easy to see how she might think that chocolate causes hyperactivity. Or how about eating a piece of chocolate and feeling more alert? Once again, you might assume that chocolate is high in caffeine. Another example is that strong desire we have for things that make us feel good, such as a great piece of chocolate. One could see how that feeling could be interpreted as a craving beyond a mere desire or want for a piece of chocolate. There are explanations, both scientific and physiological, for most of the beliefs associated with chocolate. Though examining cause and effect is an excellent method of determining facts, we are not always certain which cause has which effect, so further study is often needed. Now, in defense of these strong-held beliefs, we are learning that everyone is indeed an individual—what works for me might not work for you. For example, science shows that a low-fat diet works for some to lose weight, while others may need a little more protein to lose weight. It is all in our DNA. And each one of us is truly unique. So, again proving that a certain cause has a certain effect on you would require extensive study of your particular body physiology and metabolism.

Therefore, most general recommendations are intended to address most people, such as *eating fruits and vegetables is good for you*. But, when it comes to your beliefs and how you react and choose your foods—you are definitely one of a kind. Taking this into consideration, we are not trying to change your mind. Moreover, as we've seen, we can make quick assumptions about cause and effect and our own bodies that can be wrong. Thus, curiosity might spur you to read the explanations associated with many of chocolate's pervasive myths. Keep in mind that scientists and other experts may not agree with each other on every point when it comes to chocolate. Much of the research is conflicting, not cut and dry; the body of work falls into a gray area that makes it challenging to draw strong conclusions, particularly since many studies may rely on measures of feelings. So proponents on both sides of a debate on the myths surrounding chocolate may have some evidence. Read on and see what you think. You may find some interesting explanations to share with your fellow chocolate lovers.

SO DO WE REALLY CRAVE CHOCOLATE?

Given that chocolate is the most popular and preferred flavor among sweets, most people would say, yes, we do crave chocolate. In fact, in a recent study 91 percent of American women and 59 percent of American men reported chocolate cravings. But what is a craving and are we using the term correctly? The word *crave* is normally used loosely by most, meaning a strong desire for a certain food. On the other hand, some believe that a *craving* is the body's signal that it needs to eat something for health reasons. For example, some think that in pregnancy a craving is associated with a nutrient that the mother and baby need for their health and development. In the medical community the word *crave* has a definition that bolsters that belief: a physiological need manifested through certain appetites. In other words, your body needs a nutrient because it has grown accustomed to that nutrient or food; this type of need is generally associated with unhealthy behaviors. Or you crave a food because your body is missing a nutrient and the craving is its signal that you need to eat foods with that particular nutrient to maintain health. Though the science is ongoing, most results have shown that there is no physiological need for chocolate. In fact, most science does not support a link between a true physiological need and any particular type of food; still, there are some small studies that point to a possible link. For example, one very small study in the October 2007 issue of the *Journal of Proteome Research* showed that one's desire for chocolate may be linked to the type of bacteria living in one's digestive system. We all have bacteria in our gut that help us digest our food and may help other areas of health as well. Based on this study, those who ate chocolate every day had a different type of bacteria than those who did not. Given the size of this study, no conclusions can be drawn other than more research needs to be done to understand this better. But there could be two explanations: that a certain type of bacteria causes one to crave chocolate (or a certain nutrient found in chocolate) or that eating chocolate affects the type of bacteria in the gut.

Other studies have tested the notion that the body is craving certain nutrients or other compounds that cause the desire for chocolate. Magnesium was believed to be one of those nutrients that some may be lacking in their diets and so, given that chocolate contains magnesium, those people were suspected to crave chocolate. The study done at the University of Pennsylvania in 1994 did not find a connection, however. Another hypothesis was that caffeine and its sister compound, theobromine, were triggering such cravings. In one study at the University of Bristol, UK, in 2005, researchers did find that those consuming a drink with caffeine and theobromine enjoyed their drink more and more over time as compared to those whose drinks did not contain those compounds. The researchers concluded that these compounds, found in chocolate, may contribute to a liking for chocolate, especially the acquired taste for dark chocolate, but note that it is likely other attributes play a more important role, such as texture and taste. In trying to tease out what may be causing the desire, researchers have also fed participants the following chocolate products: cocoa powder, which contains all of chocolate's compounds and nutrients; milk chocolate, which contains all of chocolate's compounds plus conveys the enjoyment of the texture within the mouth; and white chocolate, which does not contain any of chocolate's compounds but conveys that same enjoyable melt-in-your-mouth texture. The participants were those who claimed to crave chocolate at least once a week. Interestingly, the participants' cravings were satisfied only by the milk and white chocolate, not by the cocoa powder. This study done at the University of Pennsylvania in 1994 agrees

> *Chocolate Truffle:*
> Although chocolate is not an aphrodisiac, as the ancient Aztecs believed, chocolate contains phenylethylamine (PEA), a natural substance that is reputed to stimulate the same reaction in the body as falling in love. (www.godiva.com)

with most research, that the lure of chocolate is not some special compound but instead it is the savoring of the unique sensory and flavor experience that chocolate provides.

WOMEN AND "THEIR" CHOCOLATE

Both men and women do enjoy chocolate; however, women are typically more vocal in their "needing" chocolate and their "need" often cannot be satiated by anything other than their desired chocolate treat. Furthermore, in countries that include chocolate as part of their cultural traditions, women report higher desires for chocolate than do men. So what is this special relationship that women have with chocolate? There are several potential explanations, none of which is any more or less valid than another. One school of thought is that women tend to seek high-fat, high-calorie foods around their reproductive cycle in order to build up stores to support a baby. Hormone levels may play a role. That's why prior to menstruation women will report a greater desire for

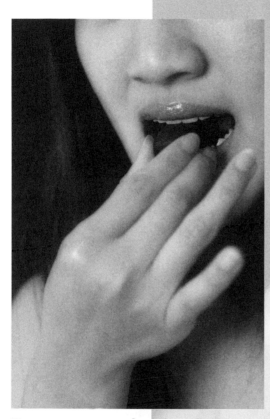

**Do women crave chocolate the most?
© Suprijono Suharjoto.
Image from BigStockPhoto.com.
Used with permission.**

Chocolate Truffle:
Chocolate contains more than 400 distinct flavor compounds, more than twice as many as any other food.

sweets, including chocolate. Interestingly, this may be culturally sensitive, as one study found this relationship held true in American women but not in Spanish women. That has led to other theories including perhaps a more emotional explanation tied to cultural practices of receiving chocolates on Valentine's Day from a "special" friend or a parent's promise of a chocolate treat for finishing dinner. It is these rituals associated with eating and receiving chocolate that help to evoke the feelings of love, romance, celebration, and comfort, and thus fuel a woman's love for chocolate. Even just the smell of chocolate may bring on these emotions; perhaps this is the reason that chocolate and cocoa bath and beauty products have become so popular.

CHOCOLATE ENHANCES THE MOOD

Contrary to the prior discussion on cravings owing to some unknown physiological need, some report that their attraction to chocolate is because of its "mood-enhancing" effects. This type of craving or attraction is often linked to a possible mood-enhancing chemical found in chocolate. So does the desire go beyond the unique combination of sweetness, smooth texture, tantalizing flavor, and enticing aroma? Perhaps it is not the chocolate itself, but instead the sensory experience, that causes a chemical reaction in our bodies that then creates our love for chocolate.

The mood-elevating benefit of chocolate is a phenomenon that the true chocolate lover has experienced, and, interestingly, may have scientific support. The sensory experience—merely looking, smelling, and tasting a good, rich piece of chocolate or chocolate dessert—can release serotonin in the brain, a feel-good hormone that can improve one's mood. Additionally, foods rich in carbohydrates, like chocolate, have been shown to reduce the stress response and keep people calm in the face of tense situations. People who tend to become depressed during such stressful times reportedly do not experience depression as often if they eat foods rich in carbohydrates. Still some believe that chocolate itself has a unique effect on mood. One study supports the idea that chocolate may act as an "anti-depressant." Researchers at the University of Wurzburg in 2006 gave thirty-seven women a snack of either an apple or a piece of chocolate. While both snacks contained carbohydrates and both elevated mood and reduced hunger, the chocolate results were stronger. So what is it about chocolate that makes us so happy? Some suggest that it does, indeed, contain specific compounds, almost

Enjoying Chocolate All Over

Similar to foods, beauty products and beauty rituals using the goodness of Mother Nature date back to ancient civilizations. Individuals as well as manufacturers have long relied on cocoa butter as a staple ingredient in their rich creams and moisturizers. In addition to cocoa butter's texture, the aroma of chocolate also has a long history in the beauty industry. However, a new trend using cocoa extracts has emerged, allowing us to benefit from potent antioxidants naturally found in the beans. Chocolate- and cocoa-based beauty products and chocolate treatments are now available at spas and salons. One of our favorites is the Hershey Spa in Hershey, Pennsylvania. Aside from enjoying the constant cocoa aroma in the air from the nearby chocolate factory or having fun at Chocolate World, one can truly experience chocolate in a whole new way, from chocolate baths to chocolate facials (all while eating chocolate or sipping rich cocoa). If Hershey, Pennsylvania, is too far from you and the trip to the spa is not realistic, we have some good news. You can create your own chocolate spa experience at home.

Enhance Your Chocolate Experience with an At-Home Chocolate Spa

First, make your own homemade chocolate bath and body products. Try the recipes that you'll find at the end of this chapter. While you make the products, play your favorite soothing music, enjoy the look of the chocolate melting in the pan and swirling in with the other ingredients, and take deep breaths, allowing the aroma to take away all distracting thoughts. Once your chocolate spa products are ready, sip a cup of hot cocoa.

Depending on your mood and to add a little pizzazz to your savory cup of cocoa, try adding one of the following ingredients:

- a little half and half to make it creamy
- a spoonful of cocoa to make it richer
- a touch of Kahlua liquor (adults only!)
- a touch of Grand Marnier liquor (again, adults only!)
- a cinnamon stick
- a peppermint stick

Then, indulge all your senses with the aroma, feel, and flavor of chocolate.

The sensory experience chocolate delivers can be replicated by no other food or drink. So in all likelihood the mood-elevating effects and even what we tend to call *cravings* for chocolate are due to its one-of-a-kind makeup that we as human beings, who appreciate sweet, melt-in-your-mouth delicacies, can savor to the fullest. Because of this unique love for chocolate, we have built chocolate into our holidays, celebrations, and good times—even those times we cherish all by ourselves.

giving it "druglike" effects. But in actuality, when chocolate is studied, the amounts of these compounds, such as alkaloids (mood-enhancing chemicals found in plants and used in medicines) or phenylethylamine (a mood-enhancing brain chemical), are so low it's unlikely that they are the reason behind chocolate's ability to engender bliss. So the most accepted explanation for why we love chocolate and why it makes us feel so good has to do more with the unique sensory experience created by the combination of rich, tantalizing flavors, and a melt-in-your-mouth texture that is rivaled by no other.

YOU MAY BE SURPRISED TO HEAR

Headaches

Migraines and headaches have long been rumored to be triggered by chocolate consumption, and surely, for some people, this may be the case. Interestingly, however, studies have not been able to demonstrate this relationship. In several studies reviewed in the September 2003 *Annals of*

Allergy and Asthma Immunology, there was no difference in the occurrence of headaches in migraine or headache sufferers after eating either chocolate or a nonchocolate-containing food. Even among those migraine sufferers who identified themselves as sensitive to chocolate as a headache trigger, researchers did not find a link. The reason that chocolate is frequently cited as sparking migraines may lie in other aspects of chocolate. Women are more likely than men to suffer from migraines and women more often report strong desires for chocolate, especially during menses. The fluctuating estrogen levels experienced with the menstrual cycle is believed to be a trigger of migraines. So

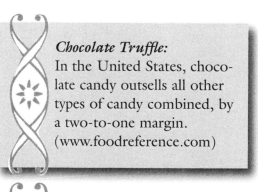

Chocolate Truffle:
In the United States, chocolate candy outsells all other types of candy combined, by a two-to-one margin. (www.foodreference.com)

the link between chocolate and migraines may be more coincidental, because of its greater consumption at a time when migraines are more likely.

Acne

Chocolate's implication in causing acne was a widespread belief in the medical community. Studies going as far back as the 1960s failed to show any link between chocolate consumption and the development of acne. A highly esteemed and extensive research review in the March 16, 1970, issue of the *Journal of the American Medical Association* on chocolate and acne stated "diet plays no role in acne treatment in most patients . . . even large amounts of chocolate have not clinically exacerbated acne." In fact, we are learning that cocoa flavanols (potent antioxidants) might even be good for your skin. As mentioned before, small studies indicate that the flavanols found in chocolate and cocoa might have a protective effect.

Hyperactivity

Anyone who has been around children excitedly receiving treats such as chocolate or candy can understand why many assume that these foods themselves cause hyperactivity. However, research has explored in depth the mistaken notion that candy and foods containing sugar, such as chocolate, are associated with hyperactivity. An extensive review of studies found that there is no relationship between consumption of sugar-containing foods and adverse effects on behavior. In addition, studies such as one from the West Virginia School of Medicine in 1996 that specifically looked at chocolate and candy failed to show any relationship between eating sugary foods and hyperactive behavior in children with and without attention-deficit hyperactivity disorder. This topic was extensively reviewed in the journal *Pediatric Nursing* in 2007, drawing the same conclusion. Basically, when people get together for a fun party or holiday where sweets are present, everyone, including the children, will get excited and "hyper."

Cavities

Preventing cavities depends on a number of factors including oral hygiene, fluoride intake, genetics, and diet. Foods containing carbohydrates may promote cavity formation. Interestingly, whether a food promotes tooth decay or not depends on how much time the food spends in the mouth. Although sweetened chocolate does contain carbohydrates, it clears the mouth relatively quickly and has not, in fact, been found to contribute to the development of cavities. One study in the *European Journal of Pediatric Dentistry*, out of Leeds, England, in 2003, investigating the response of plaque buildup from chocolates containing various levels of cocoa, found that all chocolate types had a lower effect on dental plaque than table sugar. In fact, research shows that regular brushing (twice a day) with a fluoride toothpaste has a greater impact on inhibiting the development of cavities in children than restricting sugary foods. Additionally, the British researchers found no association between consumption of chocolates and the development of cavi-

ties. Interestingly, the flavanols in cocoa may actually be good for dental health. Cocoa flavanols decrease plaque through antibacterial activity. A 2007 study at the University of Salford in Manchester, England, found that unfermented, natural cocoa powder was able to inhibit the growth of bacteria successfully. The study suggests this was due to the flavanols in the cocoa since fermented cocoa powder with a lesser amount of flavanols wasn't as effective. Additionally, a 2004 study from the University of Osaka Graduate School of Dentistry in Osaka, Japan, found that after four days of rinsing with an extract from the cacao bean shell, which is high in flavanols, while not using any other oral hygiene methods (i.e., brushing, flossing), participants had decreased bacteria and plaque on their teeth. If cocoa flavanols prevent cavities—we vote for mint chocolate–flavored toothpaste.

Caffeine

Some people do not realize that chocolate contains relatively small amounts of caffeine; a 1.4-ounce milk chocolate bar has about the same amount as a decaffeinated cup of coffee. Dark chocolate does contain more, but still much less than a cup of regular coffee.

Chocolate does, however, contain a close relative to caffeine, theobromine. Although in the same family as caffeine, theobromine has been found to have different health effects. For one, it is believed that theobromine does not have the same stimulating effect on the central nervous system as caffeine. Additionally, theobromine has been used to treat heart disease and hypertension and may suppress coughing. A recent study in 2005 by Dr. Omar S. Usmani and colleagues at Imperial College of London suggested that theobromine suppresses activity in the vagus nerve, which is the nerve that runs from the brain down to the abdomen and is responsible for coughing. In fact, theobromine has been shown to be nearly 30 percent more effective in stopping persistent coughs than the leading medicine, codeine. So you may see chocolate popping up in the cough medicine aisle as well.

Now that we've dispelled some of the modern-day myths and long-held historical beliefs about chocolate, it's obvious that no matter what one's opinion is on how chocolate affects the body, it is a topic of passion that sparks great debate. There aren't many other foods that arouse such emotion and controversy.

Chocolate Truffle:
Chocolate is dangerous to dogs because they lack the enzyme to metabolize theobromine.

Cocoa Cravings: Bath and Body

Courtesy of facts-about-chocolate.com
(http://www.facts-about-chocolate.com/chocolate-beauty-recipes.html)

Chocolate beauty recipes are easy to make and fun to give!

Chocolate Facial Recipe #1

Ingredients:

½ cup unsweetened cocoa
  powder
4 tablespoons heavy
  cream
3 teaspoons cottage
  cheese
3 teaspoons ripe avocado
¼ cup honey
3 tablespoons oatmeal
  powder

Directions:

1. Mix all ingredients
together.

2. Apply to face and leave
on for 10 minutes.

3. Dampen with warm,
moist washcloth to remove,
then apply moisturizer.

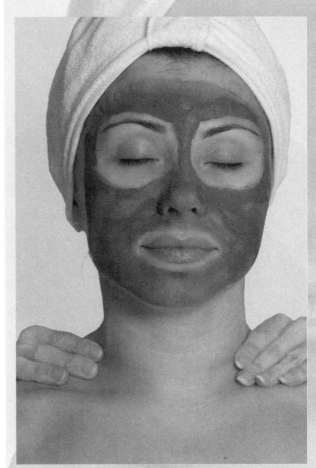

Treat yourself to a chocolate facial—cocoa
and cocoa butter are proving to be very good
for the skin. © Leah-Anne Thompson.
Image from BigStockPhoto.com.
Used with permission.

Chocolate Facial Recipe #2

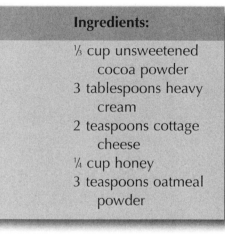

Ingredients:

⅓ cup unsweetened cocoa powder

3 tablespoons heavy cream

2 teaspoons cottage cheese

¼ cup honey

3 teaspoons oatmeal powder

Directions:

1. Mix all ingredients together.

2. Apply to face and leave on for 10 minutes.

3. Dampen with warm, moist washcloth to remove, then apply moisturizer.

Chocolate Shampoo Recipe

Ingredients:

¼ cup water
¼ cup castile soap
½ teaspoon extra virgin olive oil
½ teaspoon jojoba oil
5 drops of chocolate fragrance oil

Directions:

1. Mix all ingredients.
2. Pour shampoo into container and let stand for a few hours to thicken. Use as you would your regular shampoo.

© Mikko Pitkänen. Image from BigStockPhoto.com. Used with permission.

Chocolate Body Scrub Recipe

Ingredients:

¼ cup cocoa butter
(optional—will make a
thicker gel)
¾ cup liquid castile soap
⅛ cup coarse wheat bran or
finely ground almonds
¼ cup apricot kernel meal
1 tablespoon unsweetened
cocoa powder
2 tablespoons dark brown
sugar
1 tablespoon jojoba oil
½ tablespoon vitamin E oil
1½ teaspoon chocolate
fragrance oil

Directions:

1. Melt the cocoa butter over low heat (or at 50 percent power in the microwave) until melted. Remove from heat.

2. Add the castile soap and mix well.

3. Stir in remaining ingredients, breaking up any brown sugar clumps.

4. Pour into airtight container and let thicken for a day or two. For added freshness, store in refrigerator.

Chocolate Bath Gel Recipe

Ingredients:

½ cup water
1 package unflavored gelatin
½ cup gentle, unscented shampoo
5–10 drops chocolate fragrance oil

Directions:

1. Heat water to boiling, add gelatin, and stir until dissolved.

2. Remove from heat, then add the shampoo a little at a time until well mixed.

3. Add fragrance.

4. Pour into a clean container and refrigerate between uses. Consider adding cocoa powder for scent and extra exfoliation.

Chocolate Lip Balm Recipe

Ingredients:

3 tablespoons cocoa butter
3–4 chocolate chips
1 vitamin E capsule
¼ teaspoon almond extract
or olive oil

Directions:

1. Put cocoa butter in small, microwave-safe dish and melt in microwave.

2. Add chocolate chips and stir until melted, microwaving again if needed.

3. Add vitamin E and almond extract or olive oil. Stir very well. Store in a small, airtight container. Note: can use more chocolate chips or add cocoa powder as desired.

Mint Chocolate Lip Balm Recipe

Ingredients:

1 ounce beeswax
1 ounce cocoa butter
20–30 chocolate chips
(a handful)
2 ounces shea butter
1½ ounces olive oil
1½ ounces cocoa oil, shea
oil (or other oil)
1 ounce glycerin
10–20 drops peppermint
essential oil

Directions:

1. Melt beeswax and cocoa butter over low heat in saucepan.

2. Add chocolate chips and mix well.

3. Remove from heat and stir in shea butter and oils.

4. Put back on heat and continue stirring.

5. Add glycerin and stir.

6. Remove from heat and add essential oil. Mix well.

7. Pour into small, airtight containers. Try coconut or orange oil for variety.

Cocoa and Vanilla Lip Gloss Recipe

Ingredients:

16 teaspoons sweet
    almond or peach
    kernel oil
4 teaspoons beeswax
4 teaspoons cocoa butter
4 teaspoons honey
24 drops vanilla flavor oil
1 teaspoon vitamin F oil

Directions:

1. Over low heat in saucepan melt almond oil, beeswax, and cocoa butter, stirring occasionally.

2. Remove from heat and add honey, vanilla oil, and vitamin E. Mix well.

3. Pour into small, air-tight containers.

Makes a dozen

Chocolate Soap Recipe #1

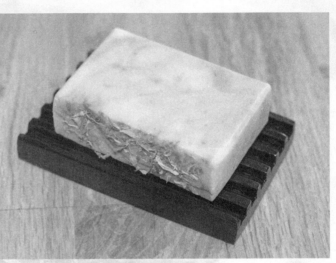

© J. B. Image from
BigStockPhoto.com.
Used with permission.

Ingredients:

½ teaspoon cocoa butter
½ teaspoon shea butter or mango
   butter
2 pounds clear coconut melt-and-
   pour soap base
1 teaspoon olive oil
½ cup goat's milk powder
2 tablespoons chocolate fragrance
   oil
1–2 tablespoons unsweetened
   cocoa powder

Directions:

1. Melt the butters and soap base over low heat in saucepan.

2. Add olive oil, then remove from heat and let cool slightly.

3. Add goat's milk powder and stir well until there are no lumps.

4. Add fragrance oil and cocoa powder until desired color and scent are reached.

5. Pour into mold. After soap hardens, release from mold.

Chocolate Soap Recipe #2

Ingredients:

1 pound white or clear
  coconut melt-and-pour
  soap base
1 pound cocoa butter
unsweetened cocoa
  powder (optional)
1 tablespoon chocolate
  fragrance oil

Directions:

1. Melt the soap base with the cocoa butter over low heat in saucepan.

2. Remove from heat and add cocoa powder for color, if desired. Stir.

3. After lumps are gone, add the oil. Pour into mold.

Cinnamon Chocolate Exfoliating Soap Recipe

Ingredients:

12 ounces coconut melt-and-pour
    soap base
15 drops cinnamon essential oil
15 drops chocolate fragrance oil
1 teaspoon unsweetened cocoa
    powder
1 tablespoon almonds, finely ground

Directions:

1. Melt soap base.
2. After melting, remove from heat and add remaining ingredients. Continue mixing gently as soap cools.
3. Pour into a large rectangular mold. Allow to set completely before removing from mold.

Chocolate and Vanilla Soap Recipe

Ingredients:

2 ounces clear coconut melt-and-pour
  soap base
½ teaspoon cocoa butter
10 drops chocolate fragrance oil
unsweetened cocoa powder
2 ounces white coconut melt-and-pour
  soap base
10 drops vanilla fragrance oil
  (or peppermint, coconut, etc.)

Directions:

1. Melt the clear soap.
2. Add cocoa butter and mix.
3. Remove from heat and mix in cocoa powder to color.
4. Let cool slightly and add chocolate fragrance oil. Pour into a mold, filling halfway. Let sit 30 minutes.
5. Melt the white soap. Remove from heat, let cool slightly, and add vanilla fragrance oil.
6. Let cool a few more minutes, then pour into mold on top of first layer. After soap hardens, release from mold.

Chocolate Orange Soap Cupcakes Recipe

Ingredients:

2 bars unperfumed cream bath soap (about 8 ounces)

1 tablespoon unsweetened cocoa powder

½ teaspoon ground cinnamon

5 teaspoons walnut oil, hazelnut oil, or almond extract

40 drops orange, peppermint, coconut, or chocolate fragrance oil

5 tablespoons mineral water or bottled water

Directions:

1. Grate the bath soap, or grind in a food processor.

2. In glass mixing bowl, mix the soap, cocoa, cinnamon, and oils.

3. Heat the water until hot but not boiling.

4. Add to the mixture and knead to form a dough.

5. Divide mixture into 4–6 portions, roll into balls, then flatten slightly.

6. Allow to dry on wax paper, about 2–3 days. Makes a nice gift when placed in a paper muffin cup, dusted with cocoa powder, and wrapped in plastic wrap.

Makes 4–6 soaps

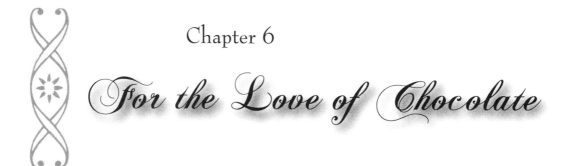

Chapter 6

For the Love of Chocolate

"Nine out of ten people like chocolate. The tenth person always lies . . ."
　—John Q. Tullius

"There is nothing better than a good friend—except a good friend with chocolate."
　—Unknown

"Chocolate is a perfect food, as wholesome as it is delicious, a beneficent restorer of exhausted power. It is the best friend of those engaged in literary pursuits."
　—Baron Justus von Liebig

CHOCOLATE AND OUR LIVES

We all have our reasons for eating chocolate—some find chocolate quietly comforting while others eat chocolate to celebrate. And some of us find any occasion the right time to enjoy a piece of chocolate. Along with a variety of reasons for eating chocolate, we all experience different effects. Some of us report feeling happy, loved, satisfied, comforted, and wanting more, while others may feel guilty or even "fat" if they eat too much.

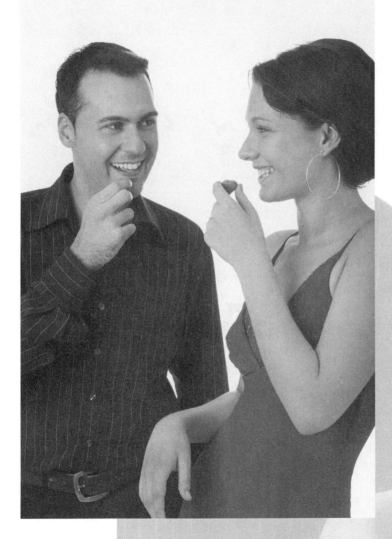

The good feelings and memories chocolate conjures are just some of the reasons this luscious treat is one of the most beloved foods for many people around the world. © Nicholas Sutcliffe. Image from BigStockPhoto.com. Used with permission.

Whatever is the outcome of consuming chocolate, deep feelings persist. Having worked in the chocolate industry for ten-plus years, we have attended several focus groups devoted to chocolate. During a focus group you sit in a room with a moderator while the marketers, product development people, and salespeople sit behind double-sided mirrors taking notes to learn what a group of individuals thinks and feels about a product, in our case, chocolate. The purpose is to help the company come up with new products and advertising campaigns. We have thus spent plenty of time contemplating and trying to understand what drives this deep passion for chocolate. While writing this book, we decided to further our understanding of the love of chocolate in a more relaxed atmosphere than that of a focus group. We had chocolate and wine socials with our friends and family—all in the name of research, of course. We created a "Chocolate Testimonials" questionnaire that was filled out during the festivities while consuming chocolate. We found that the emotional ties and feelings about chocolate have not changed over the years. In fact, answers were consistent with the hundreds of focus groups that we had attended over the years.

Chocolate is associated with love, comfort, sexiness, and indulgence. For example, one of the questions we asked was "If chocolate were an outfit what would it look like?" Answers were consistent with what we had heard before: from sexy and slinky dresses or blouses to warm pajamas or a soft robe. The rich sensual experiences of eating chocolate bring to the surface those passionate feelings that we often repress during our daily activities. One woman associated chocolate with romance and imagined "sitting in a bubble bath selecting little bits of dark chocolate from a beautiful dish." Many also reported enjoying chocolate, be it ice cream or solid chocolate, during the stillness and quiet of the night, after the children were asleep. Eating chocolate for many also conjures up those idealized carefree childhood memories. Several chocolate lovers described chocolate to be like "a sweet memory," or like "being a kid, going to play at the park," or even "a warm nap on a cold day."

Chocolate evokes not only a very personal response of having enjoyed it alone, but it is also associated with friends and family. When asked to describe their most memorable experience with chocolate, every mom told a story of time spent with her children or husband or of a wonderful moment when she was a child. Many stories included going out to eat chocolate ice cream as a family or making chocolate-dipped strawberries with the kids. Here are some of our favorites:

"My daughter was sitting on the bed with her brothers right after Halloween. She was five months old—she managed to get a chocolate bar in her mouth and lifted her head off the bed grinning ear to ear with her face absolutely covered in chocolate. I took a picture of her."

Heather Hamblen,
mother of four

"Last year my daughter was eating Hershey Kisses, the bag melted, and she was outside on our patio and started writing on the wall in chocolate."

Jennifer Mauz,
mother of one

"Our daughter, Elana, from age seven to eleven would eat Ben and Jerry's chocolate fudge brownie ice cream for dessert almost every night. Since she would find it necessary to pick out all the pieces of brownie with her hands, she absolutely could not eat it without being a complete chocolate mess—her face and hands covered in chocolate. Despite challenges and bribes to stay clean, she could never do it."

Sue Kuhl Wilson,
mother of three

"My favorite chocolate memory is my kid's first birthday cake—messy, naked baby."

Christi Petty,
mother of two

"Watching my one-year-old absolutely devour a cup of chocolate pudding, the first time he ate it, and then capturing the moment with numerous photos of his head-to-chin practically painted in chocolate, is my favorite food memory, so far."

Sarah Koenigsberg,
mother of one

"Chocolate shakes during pregnancy were my absolute favorite treat! I made my own chocolate shake by adding milk and popping it in the microwave for thirty seconds."

Julie Silhan,
mother of three

"I preferred fruit-flavored sweets to chocolate up until my first pregnancy. My husband and I were staying at a lavish hotel in Italy, on a trip celebrating the new baby-to-be, and we received these rich, indulgent Belgian chocolates every night. I was walking through the lobby one morning when the concierge called me over and offered me some extra pieces to enjoy later (for the baby, he said with a wink). From that moment on, I became a lover of chocolate. Perhaps my tastebuds changed, or perhaps each nibble of chocolate somehow takes me back to that sweet time of waiting in excited anticipation for our firstborn. I just know that something changed around that time and chocolate has remained my sweet treat of choice."

Amy Gross,
mother of three

"When I was about six or seven at summer camp I realized I would do almost anything for chocolate. Mind you, my palate was young, and I was not as particular about the type of chocolate I ate, as long as it wasn't white chocolate (this hasn't changed). Camp required swimming each day and the pool where we swam had a high diving board. I enjoyed diving off the low board regularly. Throughout the summer I had been asked to dive off the high dive, but I was too afraid. One day, one of the counselors presented a challenge . . . dive off the high dive for a Hostess Chocolate Cupcake. For the chocolate cupcake . . . I dove. The dive was well worth it — not only for the cupcake, but for a longtime appreciation of diving and for cupcakes."

Marcey Lieberman

"When I went to overnight camp, every Sunday we had a cookout and for dessert we made s'mores over the campfire. We'd break a graham cracker in half, put enough of a Hershey's chocolate bar on one side to cover the cracker, add two roasted marshmallows, and cover it with the other half of the graham cracker—yum, what a treat! As I have such wonderful memories of camp and loved the s'mores so much, I now make them over my electric stove—I just turn the burner to high and roast the marshmallows. My other favorite chocolate memory: when I was a kid, whenever we'd get a box of chocolates and I didn't like a particular one, I would give it to my father to finish for me. I guess he wasn't as picky as I was, as they never went to waste. If he wasn't around, I would gouge out a small taste of the candy from the bottom with my pinky nail and if I didn't like it I would put it back."

Susan Kolb Wilson,
mother of two,
grandmother of five

"When I was a little girl, my grandfather used to give me Hershey bars to eat—he loved them and so did I. He would offer me one if I would get rid of my chewing gum. My mother didn't like me eating candy, so she gave me chewing gum instead. I got a lot of mileage (and Hershey bars) out of manipulating this situation when we visited my grandfather."

Betty Kolb,
grandmother of three,
great-grandmother of five

"As a child, my dad would take me to Friendly's to share an all-chocolate sundae: chocolate ice cream, chocolate syrup, chocolate chips, and M&Ms. Now that he's gone I love to remember that special time together."

Rima Nachshen,
mother of two

"My favorite chocolate memory is enjoying an entire chocolate mint cake by myself after the birth of my first child. It was the only time in my life where I didn't care about the calories and just enjoyed eating my cake. I had to hide it from friends and family because I didn't want to share!"

Melissa Deutsch,
mother of three

"I got a box of Godiva Chocolate Truffles as a gift and hid them from my husband and children. Every night after everyone was in bed I would have a few and savor every bite, thinking 'this is what chocolate should taste like!'"

Ilene Fiorentino,
mother of two

"My most memorable experience with chocolate is when my husband, Jeff, and I were on the top of the Swiss Alps. We had found the perfect spot with the very best view. In our pack we pulled out a delicious bar of locally made chocolate from the town below and split a bottle of red wine. With our plastic cups filled and our taste buds drowning in rich chocolate silkiness, we watched the clouds paint themselves onto a blanket of green for hours. It was a good day."

Kara Vachon,
mother of two

Throughout history and continuing to today, chocolate is a food that evokes great passion and love. Our personal stories continue to build on a culture that started so long ago. The relics of the Aztecs and the Maya still hold the personal stories of those who created the pottery or painted their mother as she poured chocolate. And, the kings and queens who helped make chocolate so popular surely had secret stories that swirled around intrigue and chocolate. The testimonials above add to the history and lore of chocolate. Thus, the story does not end here, for this is merely a stopping point for the book. Your customs and family traditions and celebrations will lend testimony to tomorrow's relationship with chocolate. And, as such, the chocolate story continues.

We hope by delving into its rich past; discovering its health-giving potential; appreciating its mouthwatering, unique flavor notes; understanding its bounty of nutrients; and delighting in the thousands of luscious ways chocolate can be savored, you have become a true connoisseur and enthusiast of nature's gift of cacao. We have treasured the experience of taking you on this journey and wish for you a tasty life full of all of the chocolate wonder there is yet to discover.

Cocoa Cravings: Family Recipes

We wish you the joy of trying these recipes and creating your own in sampling the many textures, tastes, and richness that chocolate has to offer.

Better-Than-Sex Cake Recipe #1
Jennifer Griffith's family recipe

Ingredients:

1 cup flour
1 stick butter
½ cup chopped pecans
8 ounces cream cheese softened
1 cup Cool Whip
1 cup powdered sugar
1 small package instant vanilla
 pudding mix
1 small package instant chocolate
 pudding mix
2 cups milk

Directions:

1. Mix together flour, butter, and pecans and press into casserole dish. Bake at 350° F for 20 minutes and cool.

2. Mix together cream cheese, Cool Whip, and powdered sugar and spread over first layer.

3. Mix together vanilla and chocolate pudding mixes with milk and spread over second layer.

4. Top with more Cool Whip and grated chocolate.

Yield: 12 servings

Better-Than-Sex Cake Recipe #2
Courtesy of Heather Hamblen

Ingredients:

3 ounces unsweet-
ened chocolate
2 cups flour
1 teaspoon baking
soda
1 teaspoon salt
1½ cups sugar
⅓ cup vegetable short-
ening
1 cup sour cream
2 eggs
1 teaspoon vanilla
extract
¼ cup hot water
1 cup chocolate chips
1 jar hot fudge sauce
1 jar caramel sauce
1 tub of Cool Whip
Crushed Heath bars to
taste

Directions:

1. Preheat oven to 350° F. Grease a 9 × 13-inch pan.

2. Melt chocolate in a small cup or bowl set in simmering water, then set aside to cool.

3. Sift the flour, baking soda, salt, and sugar together in a large mixing bowl.

4. Add shortening and the sour cream and beat for about 1 minute.

5. Stir in the melted chocolate, then add the eggs, vanilla, and hot water, and beat for about 1 more minute.

6. Stir in the chocolate chips.

7. Pour the batter into prepared pan and bake for about 30 to 35 minutes or until toothpick inserted comes out clean. Remove from oven.

8. While cake is still hot, pour heated hot fudge and caramel sauce over cake. Spread to cover. Cool completely.

9. Spread Cool Whip across top of the cake and sprinkle with crushed Heath bars.

Chocolate Cake Balls
Coni Felinski's family recipe

Ingredients:

1 box chocolate cake mix
1 tub of chocolate frosting
1 container of chocolate almond bark

Directions:

1. Day 1—Bake cakes according to directions on box. Let cakes cool. Crumble cooled cake into a large bowl with tub of frosting. Form into one large ball and cool in fridge overnight.

2. Day 2—Form cake mixture into little balls and place in freezer overnight.

3. Day 3—Dip balls with spoon into melted almond bark and allow to dry. Store in loose wrap on shelf. Enjoy!

German Chocolate Cake Balls
Diane Malloy's family recipe

Ingredients:

1 box German chocolate cake mix
1 container German chocolate icing
3 ounces shredded coconut
2 packages chocolate bark candy coating

Directions:

1. Prepare cake according to package directions. Cool.

2. Crumble cake into large mixing bowl.

3. Add icing and coconut to cake and stir together well.

4. Roll mixture into small balls.

5. Melt bark candy coating in microwave according to package directions.

6. Carefully dip balls into chocolate coating and set on wax paper to harden.

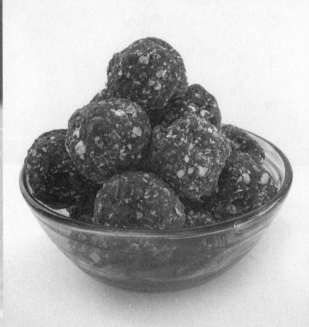

© Maree W. Image from BigStockPhoto.com. Used with permission.

Hazelnut Chocolate Chunk Cookies
Courtesy of Marcey Lieberman

Ingredients:

2¼ cups all-purpose flour

1½ cups hazelnuts, toasted and chopped coarsely

¼ teaspoon salt

1 teaspoon baking powder

1 teaspoon baking soda

2 tablespoons instant espresso powder

1 teaspoon pure vanilla extract

1 cup (2 sticks) butter, softened

1 cup packed brown sugar

1 cup sugar

2 eggs

8 ounces bittersweet chocolate chips

8 ounces block of semisweet chocolate, coarsely chopped

Directions:

1. Preheat the oven to 350° F.

2. Toast hazelnuts. Place onto a rimmed baking sheet, toast, shaking once or twice until golden (15–17 minutes). Chop half the hazelnuts coarsely and grind the other half into a powder (or purchase hazelnut flour).

3. Increase oven temperature to 375° F.

4. Cream butter.

5. Add sugar and continue whisking until light and fluffy.

6. Add vanilla.

7. Add eggs and mix on low speed.

8. In a separate bowl, whisk together flour, salt, baking soda, and ground hazel nuts.

9. Beat just until blended.

10. Stir in the chocolate.

11. Scoop batter into 1-inch balls on a parchment-lined baking sheet.

12. Bake until edges are golden, about 13–15 minutes.

13. Cool completely.

Enjoy!

Rocky Road
Courtesy of Adena Feinstein

Ingredients:

10-ounce bag of mini marshmallows
8–10-ounce can of honey-roasted peanuts
16-ounce bag of raisins
72 ounces of semisweet chocolate morsels

Directions:

1. Mix marshmallows, raisins, and peanuts together in a big mixing bowl.

2. In a separate microwave-safe bowl, melt chocolate in the microwave, 1–2 minutes at a time. Make sure you mix periodically as you melt the chocolate so it doesn't burn.

3. Cover your marshmallow mixture completely with the melted chocolate.

4. Use a tablespoon to dollop out your mixture onto ungreased cookie sheets. Put in freezer to harden.

5. After they are hard, store in Ziploc bags in the freezer. Take out of freezer one hour before serving.

Chocolate Chip Fun and Friends Cake
by Mrs. Michael S. Fayne (Compliments of Chocoholic.com—
your connection to the world of Premium Chocolates)

Ingredients:

1 stick (8 tablespoons,
    or ½ cup) butter,
    softened
1 cup sugar
2 eggs
¼ teaspoon vanilla
1⅓ cups flour
1⅓ teaspoons baking
    powder
1 teaspoon baking soda
¾ teaspoon cinnamon
1 cup sour cream
1½ cups (12 ounces)
    good-quality dark
    chocolate chips or
    chopped chocolate
    (use a bit less for a
    less rich cake)

Directions:

1. Preheat oven to 350° F, and prepare a Bundt® style pan or tube pan with shortening and flour.

2. Cream butter and sugar together (in a bowl large enough for a one-cake cake batter).

3. Beat in eggs and vanilla, stir well.

4. Sift in flour, baking powder, baking soda, and cinnamon. Stir quite well.

5. Mix in sour cream (or acidulated milk or yogurt), stirring well.

6. Add chocolate chips or chopped chocolate, and stir just to fully incorporate.

7. Bake at 350° F for 35 to 40 minutes. Test with toothpick (should be clean but not overly dry)—check at the earlier time, as ovens can vary.

8. Cool and turn over onto cake plate. Don't worry, this is not a high-rising cake. And the chocolate chips will most likely sink to the bottom of the pan, so when you invert it, prepare for gooey, chocolatey fun.

Chocolate and Macadamia Fudge

*by Jessica Claire Bondaruk (Compliments of Chocoholic.com—
your connection to the world of Premium Chocolates)*

Directions:

1. Spread the macadamia nuts on an oven tray. Roast the nuts under a pre-heated broiler. Roast 2–3 minutes or until the nuts are golden brown. Shake the tray regularly so the nuts are roasted evenly.

2. Allow the nuts to cool slightly, then chop them using a large knife.

3. Place the condensed milk, dark chocolate, and butter in a medium pan. Stir the mixture with a wooden spoon over low heat until the chocolate and butter have melted and the mixture is smooth.

4. Remove the pan from the heat and stir in the roasted chopped nuts; mix well.

5. Spread the mixture evenly into an 8 x 8-inch pan that has been lined with wax paper. Smooth the top of the fudge and refrigerate it for at least 3 hours or until it has set.

Ingredients:

6 ounces macadamia nuts
1 can (14-ounce size) sweetened
    condensed milk
18 ounces dark chocolate
    (chopped)
2 tablespoons butter
2 ounces white chocolate
    (melted)

6. When the fudge has set, turn it out of the pan and remove the wax paper. Cut the fudge into squares or triangles. You may need to use a warm knife.

7. Place the melted white chocolate in a plastic bag, snip a small hole in a corner, and drizzle a little chocolate over the top of each piece.

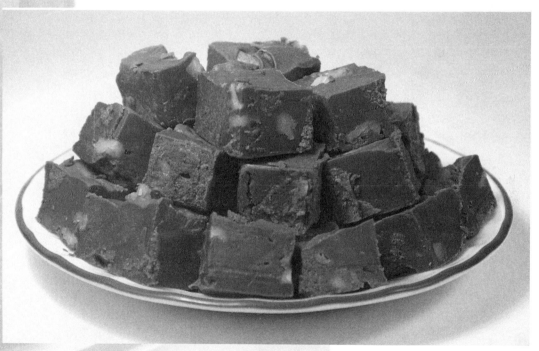

© Kathy Libby. Image from BigStockPhoto.com. Used with permission.

Brownie Surprise
Courtesy of Elana Wilson

Ingredients:

Any boxed brownie recipe, prepared in an 8 x 8-inch pan
1 cup of marshmallow fluff
1½ cups chocolate chips
¾ cup Rice Krispies
2 tablespoons peanut butter

Directions:

1. Prepare brownies according to package directions.

2. Once brownies are cooled, spread a thick layer of marshmallow fluff on brownies.

3. Melt chocolate chips in a covered microwave-safe container on high for 1½ minutes.

4. Mix Rice Krispies and peanut butter into melted chocolate and then spread mixture on top of layer of fluff. Cool in refrigerator. Best served cool.

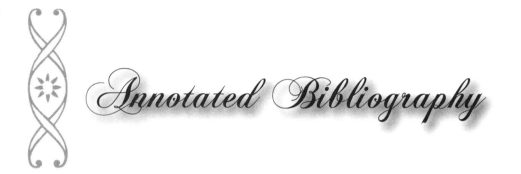

Annotated Bibliography

Brenner, Joel Glenn. *The Emperors of Chocolate: Inside the Secret World of Hershey and
Mars*. New York: Random House, 1999.

Coe, Michael D., and Sophie D. Coe. *The
True History of Chocolate*. New York:
Thames & Hudson, 1996.

Cortes, H. Hernan. *Cortes: Letters from
Mexico*. 1519. New Haven, CT: Yale
University Press, 1986.

Diaz del Castillo, B. *The Conquest of New Spain,
1560–1568*. New York: Penguin, 1983.

http://www.exploratorium.edu/exploring/
exploring_chocolate/choc_5.html.

http://www.fieldmuseum.org/Chocolate/
history.html.

www.allchocolate.com and the Hershey
Company

www.chocolateusa.org and the Chocolate
Manufacturers Association

www.ghirardelli.com

www.godiva.com

www.lindt.com

www.mars.com

www.nestle.com

www.scharffenberger.com

RESEARCH STUDIES

Buijsse, B., E. J. Feskens, F. J. Kok, and D. Kromhout. "Cocoa Intake, Blood Pressure, and Cardiovascular Mortality: The Zutphen Elderly Study." *Archives of Internal Medicine* 166 (2006): 411–17.

Chaitman, B. R. "Comments and Discussion on the Cocoa-Platelet Presentation." *Journal of Cardiovascular Pharmacology* 47, supp. 2 (2006): S206–S209.

Dillinger, T. L., and L. E. Grivetti. "Food of the Gods: Cure for Humanity? A Cultural History of the Medicinal and Ritual Use of Chocolate." *Journal of Nutrition* 130 (2000): 2057S–2072S.

Dinges, D. F. "Cocoa Flavanols, Cerebral Blood Flow, Cognition and Health: Going Forward." *Journal of Cardiovascular Pharmacology* 47 (2006): S221–S223.

Engler, M. B., and M. M. Engler. "The Emerging Role of Flavonoid-Rich Cocoa and Chocolate in Cardiovascular Health and Disease." *Nutrition Reviews* 64, no. 3 (2006): 109–18.

Farouque, H., M. Leung, S. A. Hope, M. Baldi, C. Schechter, J. D. Cameron, and I. T. Meredith. "Acute and Chronic Effects of Flavanol-Rich Cocoa on Vascular Function in Subjects with Coronary Artery Disease. A Randomized, Double-Blind, Placebo-Controlled Study." *Clinical Science (London)* 111, no. 1 (2006): 71–80.

Ferri, C., D. Grassi, and G. Grassi. "Cocoa Beans, Endothelial Function and Aging: An Unexpected Friendship?" *Journal of Hypertension* 24 (2006): 1471–74.

Fisher, N. D., F. A. Sorond, and N. K. Hollenberg. "Cocoa Flavanols and Brain Perfusion." *Journal of Cardiovascular Pharmacology* 47 (2006): S210–S214.

Francis, S. T., K. Head, P. G. Morris, and I. A. Macdonald. "The Effect of Flavanol-Rich Cocoa on the fMRI Response to a Cognitive Task in Healthy Young People." *Journal of Cardiovascular Pharmacology* 47 (2006): S215–S220.

Grassi, D., C. Lippi, S. Necozione, G. Desideri, and C. Ferri. "Short-Term Administration of Dark Chocolate Is Followed by a Significant Increase in Insulin Sensitivity and a Decrease in Blood Pressure in Healthy Persons." *American Journal of Clinical Nutrition* 81 (2004): 611–14.

Grassi, D., S. Necozione, C. Lippi, G. Croce, L. Valeri, P. Pasqualetti, G. Desideri, J. B. Blumberg, and C. Ferri. "Cocoa Reduces Blood Pressure and Insulin Resistance and Improves Endothelium-Dependent Vasodilation in Hypertensives." *Hypertension* 46, no. 2 (2005): 398–405.

Heinrich, U., K. Neukam, H. Tronnier, H. Sies, and W. Stahl. "Long-Term Ingestion of High Flavanol Cocoa Provides Photoprotection against UV-Induced Erythema and Improves Skin Condition in Women." *Journal of Nutrition* 136 (2006): 1565–69.

Heptinstall, S., J. May, S. Fox, C. Kwik-Uribe, and L. Zhao. "Cocoa Flavanols and Platelet and Leukocyte Function: Recent In Vitro and Ex Vivo Studies in Healthy Adults." *Journal of Cardiovascular Pharmacology* 47, supp. 2 (2006): S197–S205.

Hermann F., L. E. Speiker, F. Ruschitzka, I. Sudano, M. Hermann, C. Binggeli, T. F. Luscher, W. Riesen, G. Noll, and R. Corti. "Dark Chocolate Improves Endothelial and Platelet Function." *Heart* 92 (2006): 119–20.

Hollenberg, N. "Vascular Action of Cocoa Flavanols in Humans: The Roots of the Story." *Journal of Cardiovascular Pharmacology* 47 (2006): S99–S102.

Holt, R. R., D. D. Schramm, C. L. Keen, S. A. Lazarus, and H. Schmitz. "Flavonoid-Rich Chocolate and Platelet Function." *Journal of the American Medical Association* 287 (2002): 2212–13.

Jordain, C., G. Tenca, A. Deguercy, P. Troplin, and D. Poelman. "In-Vitro Effects of Polyphenols from Cocoa and Betasitosterol on the Growth of Human Prostate Cancer and Normal Cells." *European Journal of Cancer Prevention* 15 (2006): 353–61.

Kay, C. D., P. M. Kris-Etherton, and S. G. West. "Effects of Antioxidant-Rich Foods on Vascular Reactivity: Review of the Clinical Evidence." *Current Atherosclerosis Report* 8 (2006): 510–22.

Kenny, T. P., C. L. Keen, H. H. Schmitz, and M. E. Gershwin. "Immune Effects of Cocoa Procyanidin Oligomers on Peripheral Blood Mononuclear Cells." *Experiments in Biological Medicine* 232 (2007): 294–300.

Lee, K. W., J. K. Kundu, S. O. Kim, K. Chun, H. J. Lee, and Y. Surh. "Cocoa Polyphenols Inhibit Phorbol Ester-Induced Superoxide Anion Formation in Cultured HL-60 Cells and Expression of Cyclooxygenase-2 and Activation of NF-kB and MAPKs in Mouse Skin In Vivo." *Journal of Nutrition* 126 (2006): 1150–55.

Matsumoto, M., M. Tsuji, J. Okuda, H. Sasaki, K. Nakano, K. Osawa, S. Shimura, and T. Ooshima. "Inhibitory Effects of Cacao Bean Husk Extract on Plaque Formation In Vitro and In Vivo." *European Journal of Oral Science* 112, no. 3 (2004): 249–52.

McCullough, M. L., K. Chevaux, L. Jackson, M. Preston, G. Martinez, H. H. Schmitz, C. Coletti, H. Campos, and N. K. Hollenberg. "Hypertension, the Kuna, and the Epidemiology of Flavanols." *Journal of Cardiovascular Pharmacology* 47 (2006): S103–S109.

Mink, P. J., C. G. Scrafford, L. M. Barraj, L. Harnack, C. P. Hong, J. A. Nettleton, and D. R. Jacobs. "Flavonoid Intake and Cardiovascular Disease Mortality: A Prospective Study in Postmenopausal Women." *American Journal of Clinical Nutrition* 85 (2007): 895–909.

Murphy, K. J., A. K. Chronopoulos, I. Singh, et al. "Dietary Flavanols and Procyanidin Oligomers from Cocoa (*Theobroma cacao*) Inhibit Platelet Function." *American Journal of Clinical Nutrition* 77 (2003): 1466–73.

Nettleton, J. A., L. J. Harnack, C. G. Scrafford, P. J. Mink, L. M. Barraj, and D. R. Jacobs. "Dietary Flavonoids and Flavonoid-Rich Foods Are Not Associated with Risk of Type 2 Diabetes in Postmenopausal Women." *Journal of Nutrition* 136 (2006): 3039–45.

Neukam, K., W. Stahl, H. Tronnier, H. Sies, and U. Heinrich. "Consumption of Flavanol-Rich Cocoa Acutely Increases Microcirculation in Human Skin." *European Journal of Nutrition* 46 (2007): 53–56.

Ochodnicky, P., R. H. Henning, R. van Dokkum, and D. de Zeeuw. "Microalbuminuria and Endothelial Dysfunction: Emerging Targets for Primary Prevention of End-Organ Damage." *Journal of Cardiovascular Pharmacology* 47 (2006): S151–S162.

Pearson, D., T. Paglieroni, D. Rein, et al. "The Effects of Flavanol-Rich Cocoa and Aspirin on Ex Vivo Platelet Function." *Thrombosis Research* 106 (2002): 191–97.

Rein, D., T. G. Paglieroni, D. Rein, T. Wun, et al. "Cocoa Inhibits Platelet Activation and Function." *American Journal of Clinical Nutrition* 72 (2000): 30–35.

Schroeter, H., C. Heiss, J. Balzar, P. Kleinbongard, C. Keen, N. Hollenberg, H. Sies, C. Kwik-Uribe, H. Schmitz, and M. Kelm. "(-)-Epicatechin Mediates Beneficial Effects of Flavanol-Rich Cocoa on Vascular Function in Humans." *PNAS* 103 (2006): 1024–29.

Selmi, C., T. K. Mao, C. L. Keen, H. H. Schmitz, and M. E. Gershwin. "The Anti-inflammatory Properties of Cocoa Flavanols." *Journal of Cardiovascular Pharmacology* 47 (2006): S163–S171.

Singh, I., H. Quinn, M. Mok, R. J. Southgate, A. H. Turner, D. Li, A. J. Sinclair, and J. A. Hawley. "The Effect of Exercise and Training Status on Platelet Activation: Do Cocoa Polyphenols Play a Role?" *Platelets* 17, no. 6 (2006): 361–67.

Smullen, J., G. A. Koutsou, H. A. Foster, A. Zumbé, and D. M. Storey. "The Antibacterial Activity of Plant Extracts Contyaining Polyphenols against *Streptococcus mutans*." *Caries Research* 41, no. 5 (2007): 342–49.

Steffen, Y., T. Schewe, and H. Sies. "Myeloperoxidase-Mediated LDL Oxidation and Endothelial Cell Toxicity of Oxidized LDL: Attenuation by (-)-epicatechin." *Free Radical Research* 40 (2006): 1076–85.

Sudano, I., L. E. Spieker, F. Hermann, A. Flammer, R. Corti, G. Noll, and T. F. Luscher. "Protection of Endothelial Function: Targets for Nutritional and Pharmacological Interventions." *Journal of Cardiovascular Pharmacology* 47 (2006): S136–S150.

Taubert, D., R. Roesen, and E. Schomig. "Effect of Cocoa and Tea Intake on Blood Pressure: A Meta-Analysis." *Archives of Internal Medicine* 167, no. 7 (April 9, 2007): 626–34.

Tomaru, M., H. Takano, N. Osakabe, A. Yasuda, K. Inoue, R. Yanagisawa, T. Ohwatari, and H. Uematsu. "Dietary Supplementation with Cacao Liquor Proanthocyanidins Prevents Elevation of Blood Glucose Levels in Diabetic Obese Mice." *Nutrition* 23, no. 4 (2007): 351–55.

Vinson, J. A., J. Proch, P. Bose, S. Muchler, P. Taffera, D. Shuta, N. Samman, and G. A. Agbor. "Chocolate Is a Powerful Ex Vivo and In Vivo Antioxidant, an Antiatherosclerotic Agent in an Animal Model and a Significant Contributor to Antioxidants in the European and American Diets." *Journal of Agricultural Food Chemistry* 54 (2006): 8071–76.

Vlachapoulos, C., N. Alexopoulos, and C. Stefanadis. "Effect of Dark Chocolate on Arterial Function in Healthy Individuals: Cocoa Instead of Ambrosia?" *Current Hypertension Report* 8 (2006): 205–11.

Wang-Polagruto, J. F., A. C. Villablanca, J. A. Polagruto, L. Lee, R. R. Holt, H. R. Schrader, J. L. Ensunsa, F. M.

Steinberg, H. H. Schmitz, and C. L. Keen. "Chronic Consumption of Flavanol-Rich Cocoa Improves Endothelial Function and Decreases Vascular Cell Adhesion Molecule in Hypercholesterolemic Postmenopausal Women. *Journal of Cardiovascular Pharmacology* 47, supp. 2 (2006): S177–S186.

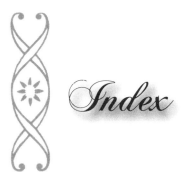

Index